Advanced
Spiritual Intimacy

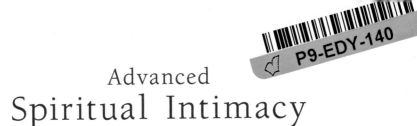

"Stuart Sovatsky's *Advanced Spiritual Intimacy* is a tour de force. He takes us beyond the texts to demonstrate how the ancient path of spiritual growth may extend across a whole lifetime. This book expands our Western hermeneutic of tantra toward engendering a paradigm shift in the methodology for all who have been teaching its ways for years or decades. And as years and lifecycles unfold for persons of all walks of life, this study may help to honor the depths of Indian marriage from the depths of Sanātana Dharma itself."

PURUSHOTTAMA BILIMORIA, PH.D.;
CHANCELLOR'S SCHOLAR, UC BERKELEY; POST-DOCTORATE FELLOW,
OXFORD UNIVERSITY; EDITOR IN CHIEF OF *SOPHIA* JOURNAL

"This book reveals tantra's most central and powerful aspect: converting sexual energy into a higher, consciousness-altering vitality. Stuart Sovatsky's vast knowledge and four decades of practice of tantra yoga and his lifelong work as a relationship therapist is a perfect combination for his book *Advanced Spiritual Intimacy*. A must read for all who aspire to a spiritual way of life and are wondering just where sex fits in."

GEORG FEUERSTEIN, PH.D., AUTHOR OF *SACRED SEXUALITY*, AND
BRENDA FEUERSTEIN, AUTHOR OF *TRADITIONAL YOGA STUDIES* AND
DIRECTOR OF THE GEORG FEUERSTEIN INNER FREEDOM PROJECT

"*Advanced Spiritual Intimacy* is an excellent book that will help couples and individuals to grow and master themselves."

FRÉDÉRIC LUSKIN, PH.D., AUTHOR OF *FORGIVE FOR GOOD* AND
DIRECTOR OF THE STANFORD UNIVERSITY FORGIVENESS PROJECTS

"Few people are as well positioned as Stuart Sovatsky to contribute to the West's understanding of yoga and tantra, and he has done so with *Advanced Spiritual Intimacy*. This book adds a new dimension and another level to the understanding of our ultimate potential."

PHILIP GOLDBERG, AUTHOR OF *AMERICAN VEDA*

"Through decades of pioneering service projects, writings, and his kirtans arousing of Kundalini, Stuart has uplifted the academic and spiritual landscape of the West. For those who long to meet a lifelong yogi, master, beloved of Lord Shiva, you will find such a one in the pages of *Advanced Spiritual Intimacy*."

SWAMI ADI NARAYAN, AUTHOR OF
THE BELOVED: A SONG OF ETERNAL LOVE

"Sovatsky's work brings the depths of India's spiritual path of marriage and family love to the Western world in keeping with India's core vision of Vasudhaiva kutumbakam—the world is indeed one Family—and reveals the devotional dimension of yoga in the truest voice of the Indian spiritual soul."

SUNIL SAINI, PH.D., PRESIDENT OF
INDIAN ASSOCIATION OF HEALTH, RESEARCH, AND WELFARE

"The extent of Sovatsky's knowledge is breathtaking. He makes an important and persuasive reframing of Brahmacharya as an 'inner marriage' rather than celibacy, with yoga as its own love affair with prana. He completely transforms what is currently understood as 'practicing yoga' and provides a fresh way of re-envisioning intimacy for anyone on a spiritual path."

IRA ISRAEL, MARRIAGE AND FAMILY THERAPIST AND
YOGA TEACHER/THERAPIST

"Sovatsky guides us with a master's hands to open the portals of devotional worship in yoga and in love. His book is a tour de force, beckoning lovers deeper into the seed mysteries of devotion and worship."

TINA M. BENSON, M.A., TRANSPERSONAL/JUNGIAN-ORIENTED COACH
AND FOUNDER/CREATOR OF THE SOUL SPEAKS PROJECT

"The Age of Aquarius begins right now with Stuart Sovatsky's new sexual (r)evolution. Get out your surfboards and anchor yourself on the crest of the wave with *Advanced Spiritual Intimacy*. Don't forget to enjoy the ride!"

LISA PAUL STREITFELD, CULTURAL CRITIC/PHILOSOPHER,
HUFFINGTON POST ARTS

"Stuart Sovatsky's *Advanced Spiritual Intimacy* bravely walks the cutting edge of tantra and blasts us open into spirit consciousness, while enlivening us to the potentiality of matter and flesh."

KATIE SILCOX, AUTHOR OF
HEALTHY HAPPY SEXY: AYURVEDA WISDOM FOR MODERN WOMEN

Advanced Spiritual Intimacy

The Yoga of
Deep Tantric Sensuality

Stuart Sovatsky, Ph.D.

Destiny Books
Rochester, Vermont • Toronto, Canada

Destiny Books
One Park Street
Rochester, Vermont 05767
www.DestinyBooks.com

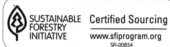

Text stock is SFI certified

Destiny Books is a division of Inner Traditions International

Originally published in 1994 by Destiny Books under the title *Passions of Innocence: Tantric Celibacy and the Mysteries of Eros*
Published in 1999 by Park Street Press under the title *Eros, Consciousness, and Kundalini: Deepening Sensuality through Tantric Celibacy and Spiritual Intimacy*

Library of Congress Cataloging-in-Publication Data
Sovatsky, Stuart, 1949–
 [Passions of innocence]
 Advanced spiritual intimacy : the yoga of deep tantric sensuality / Stuart Sovatsky. — Third edition.
  pages cm
 Includes bibliographical references and index.
 ISBN 978-1-62055-264-3 (paperback) — ISBN 978-1-62055-278-0 (e-book)
 1. Celibacy—Tantrism. 2. Kundalini. 3. Tantrism—Doctrines. 4. Sex—Religious aspects—Tantrism. I. Title.
 BL1283.852.S684 2014
 294.5'447—dc23
                                                                2013041057

Printed and bound in the United States by Lake Book Manufacturing, Inc.
The text stock is SFI certified. The Sustainable Forestry Initiative₀ program promotes sustainable forest management.

10 9 8 7 6 5 4 3 2 1

Text design and layout by Virginia Scott Bowman
This book was typeset in Garamond premier Pro and Berkeley Oldstyle with Garamond Premier Pro and Gill Sans used as display typefaces

Digital artwork photography for prologue images by Will Cloughley, Sondra Slade, Vera Vasey, Stuart Sovatsky

To send correspondence to the author of this book, mail a first-class letter to the author c/o Inner Traditions • Bear & Company, One Park Street, Rochester, VT 05767, and we will forward the communication, or contact the author directly at **stuartcs1@comcast.net** or through his website **http://home.jps.net/~stuartcs**.

For Lillian, Jacob, David, Ida, Bill, Oscar,

Anna, Samuel, Anna . . .

Contents

Acknowledgments   xi

PROLOGUE   Urdhvaretas: Yoga's Path of Complete
Maturation of Ensouled, Engendered Bodies   1

1   Everything Will Change   15

A Most Unusual Invitation   15

Awakening Dormant Seed Potentials   17

Urdhvaretas First Bursts in the Modern West   22

Reenvisioning Family Life   29

2   Entering the Mystery: Moving from
Cynical Certainty to Spiritual Intimacies   32

Something Hidden Is Going On   32

Five Degrees of Approach   34

3   Shared-Gender Mystery   51

Male and Female as Starting Points   52

Gender Is the Sharing of Mystery   53

Gender Awe   60

Gender Worship   61

The Prosthesis of an Owned Sexuality   64

Homosexual Mystery   68

4 Purposeful Urdhvaretas   **70**

Who Chooses Urdhvaretas?   71

Why You Might Choose Brahmacharya   74

Beginning and Setting a Time Frame   81

Considerations of Personality and Mystery   83

5 Yogic Anatomy and Transformation of the Ars Erotica Body   **85**

The Subtle Bodies   85

The Chakras   90

Transforming Passion into Divine Rapture   101

Meditative Knowing   105

6 Commitment and Marriage as Grihastha Mysteries   **112**

Lifelong Commitment: The Crux of Finitude   121

To Stay or to Leave?   124

Viyoga (Hidden Unions) and Spoken Passion   126

The Erotic Freedom of Belonging   130

7 The Passions and Mysteries of Fertility   **132**

Procreative Wonders   133

Meditation: Retas Mysteries   134

Creating New Life   140

Procreation and the Shared-Gender Mystery   143

Sharing a Home with Mystery   145

Ars Erotica Facts of Life for Teenagers   146

8 Within the Intimus: The Myriad Inner Empathic Spaces (IES)   **153**

Sixty-four Intimate Spaces of Ars Erotica   156

9 Communication Yoga   167

Twenty-one Verbal Asanas of Creative
Communication for Couples   169

10 Relational Worship   175

Ritual Worship of Mystery   188

This and That   190

Profundity within Simplicity   195

11 Hatha Yoga as Ars Erotica   198

Bandhas and Mudras   199

Asanas   202

Chair and Bed Yoga   214

Family Practice Ideas   215

Partnered Practices   215

Sahaja Yoga   224

12 Sringara Rasa   228

Suggestive Ambiguities of Twilight Teachings
Reveal, Conceal, and Protect the Intimus   231

Beyond Protective Ambiguities and Scholarly
Demystifying Certainties into the Sacred Intimus   235

13 Brahmacharya: Solo Intimacy with the Source   240

The Heights   244

The Saint   245

Elder Sannyasa, Letting Go   247

Afterword   249

Glossary   251

Notes   260

Bibliography   264

Index   282

Acknowledgments

This work would not be possible without the lifelong dedication of innumerable yogis, particularly L. Lakulisha, Sri Thirumoolar, Sri Atmarama, S. Kripalvananda, Amrit Desai, Umesh Baldwin, Vinit Muni, Rajasri Muni, Sri Sri Ravi Shankar, Adi-ji Narayan, Adi-ji Ananda, and Baba Hari Dass;

The academic support of Michel Foucault, Robert Thurman, Rajiv Malhotra, Sangeetha Menon, Yanez Drnovsec, Maja Milcinski, Carl Becker, David Gray, Dr. Usha Ram (University of Pune), Bal Ram Singh, David Frawley, Arindham Chakravarty, Ian Whicher, Victor Preller, William Broad, Vladimir Maykov (responsible for the Russian edition), Motilal Banarsidass (responsible for the Indian edition), T. V. Gopal (for inclusion in *Proceedings of Facets of Consciousness Conference*, Hyderabad), Diego Pignatelli (responsible for the Italian edition), Meji Singh, Ralph Metzner, Karl Kracklauer, Harold Streitfeld, Myron McClelland, Jim Ryan, and Wayne Richards;

The support of my writing efforts by Miles Vich, *Yoga Journal* U.S./Russia, Georg and Brenda Feuerstein, Craig Comstock, Marcie Boucouvalas, Keith Hoeller;

The illustrations of Alex Laurant, digitized photography of Will Cloughley and Sondra Slade, and the calligraphy of Kartik Patel and S. Chakravarty;

The many people whom I interviewed and thousands of clinical clients;

The personal support of my life partner, V. Vasey, who helped me feel every word, as well as K. Wray, Erich Gottlieb, Helen Palmer, Leland Meister, Cheryl Whyatt, Doris Warner, Peter Sutherland, Tina Benson, Ania Fizyta, A. D. H., C. F., K. J. R., K. P., M. S., Rupa, Carla King, Greg Bogart, Andrew, Maria, B. Vadhi, Naomi and Noah Groeschel, Jonathan Reynolds, Lauren Gonzalez, Leslie Combs, Purushottama Bilimoria, Zana Marovic, and Harold Johnson;

The staff of Insight Counseling and Blue Oak Counseling and my students at the California Institute of Integral Studies and John F. Kennedy University;

The Society for the Scientific Study of Sex, the World Congress of Sexology, World Congress on Psychology and Spirituality, World Association of Vedic Studies, Thirteenth Congress on Vedanta, the Association for Transpersonal Psychology, the Association of Humanistic Psychology, Shruti, Eurotas, Axis Mundi, S. Doroganich and my Russian students;

Carole DeSanti, my first editor from erstwhile E. P. Dutton, and the attentive first edition copyediting of Jill Mason;

The enthusiasm and wise publishing support of the team at Inner Traditions/Destiny Books: Jamaica Burns Griffin, Nancy Yeilding, and Jeanie Levitan for their masterful editing on this new edition; Jon Graham, Leslie Colket, Lee Wood, Anna Chapman, and publisher Ehud Sperling for their support of my work; the new edition design and layout by Virginia Scott Bowman and indexing by Brenda Feuerstein; and

The insightful editorial contributions of friend and colleague, Dan Joy, who brought sensitivity and acumen to the project.

Urdhvaretas

Yoga's Path of Complete Maturation of Ensouled, Engendered Bodies

As a juvenile probation officer, social worker, and marriage and family therapist since 1972, I have worked with three generations of individuals, couples, and families, from tragically locked-up teens going awry in the sad chaos of broken homes (both wealthy and impoverished), to thirty- and forty-year-olds spreading their hopes for love among two or three simultaneous, polyamorous or serial-monogamy partners, to the ever more numerous and grayer, fifty- and sixty-year-olds on their third go-around, living alone, away from their "previous families" and skittishly Internet dating, having real or Facebook affairs with married persons or laptop relationships with "live" porn stars.

Thus, over these past forty years, I have seen ample evidence of a widespread need for more holistic approaches to human sexuality and intimate relationships than what Freud and his scions gave to my profession and to all us "moderns." Indeed, a whole new post-Freudian psychology is needed that revives the heart and soul of romantic-erotic love itself.

I found just such a psychology in the yogic, lifelong developmental path known as *urdhvaretas*—the complete blossoming (*urdhva,* up-growing) of all human seed potentials (*retas*)—an ancient yogic tradition with abundant offerings that speak to many aspects of our modern distress, especially in the realms of our most important relationships.

Urdhvaretas is the living infinity of life's wild genetic diversity. It offers depths of meaning and feeling and consciousness so profound, ecstatic, and creative that only Sanskrit terms can truly name them. The tradition of urdhvaretas encompasses tumescences and orgasms unknown even to us liberated moderns, and loves and marriages that easily last a lifetime or two or three—the kind of relationships that support unbroken family lineages generation upon generation. With urdhvaretas, there is always another realm of seeds-within-seeds-within-seeds.

Urdhvaretas began when we each were merely "a glint of passion" flashing in the first attractions between our parents-to-be (and in their parents and in theirs). This up-growing passion became more embodied through their erotic union, more so via our conception and gestation, and even more so via the fertility-bestowing puberty of our own adolescence. But in the urdhvaretas developmental schema, the maturation of body-mind-heart-soul continues at the same dramatic level of intensity through a lifelong series of adult puberties. As with teenaged puberty, they transform identity, sense of life purpose, and erotic bodily capacities for lovemaking. These adult puberties are as yet unmapped in the West, with "kundalini* awakening" just beginning to enter the wider Western discourse. The maturations within this complete "up-blossoming" of the seed potentials include bodily secretions, tumescences, and modes of orgasm, not only beyond Freudian sex-liberation theories, but largely unknown even within the "neo-tantric sex" scene.

In his book *The History of Sexuality* the brilliant social historian Michel Foucault (1926–1984) makes a distinction that offers a useful

---

Kundalini is intelligent Mother energy that guides all embryological body-creation and then "goes to sleep" at the base of the newborn's spine, but—with the requisite practices—can reawaken to fully embodied enlightenment. This and other Sanskrit terms used in the book can be found with their definitions in the glossary at the back of the book, for your ready reference.

key to understanding the blissful urdhvaretas possibilities, open to us all, revealed in this book. He identifies "two great procedures for producing the truth of sex": *ars erotica* and *scientia sexualis*. Ars erotica is "the erotic art" that numerous societies—"China, Japan, India, Rome, the Arabo-Moslem societies"—endowed themselves with. Scientia sexualis is the term he uses to refer to both the Roman Catholic Church's moralistic, marriage-only, rhythm-method-only type of erotic "truths" as well as the "scientific truths" and psychoanalytic theory of the sex drive, the function of the orgasm, and so on, and the sexual liberation made possible by safe contraceptive/abortion technologies. (The images on the following pages provide a visual comparison of scientia sexualis versus ars erotica.*) Foucault elaborates the transforming truth to be gained from ars erotica:

> In the erotic art, truth is drawn from pleasure itself, understood as a practice and accumulated as experience; pleasure is not considered in relation to an absolute law of the permitted and the forbidden, nor by reference to a criterion of utility, but first and foremost in relation to itself; it is experienced as pleasure, evaluated in terms of its intensity, its specific quality, its duration, its reverberations in the body and the soul. Moreover, this knowledge must be deflected back into the sexual practice itself, in order to shape it as though from within and amplify its effects. In this way, there is formed a knowledge that must remain secret, not because of an element of infamy that might attach to its object, but because of the need to hold it in the greatest reserve, since according to the tradition, it would lose its effectiveness and its virtue by being divulged. . . .
>
> The effects of this masterful art, which are considerably more generous than the spareness of its prescriptions would lead one to imagine, are said to transfigure the one fortunate enough to receive its privileges: an absolute mastery of the body, a singular bliss, obliviousness to time and limits, the elixir of life, the exile of death and its threats.[1]

---

*For a gallery of additional images that accompany the text, please see home.jps .net/~stuartcs/about09.html.

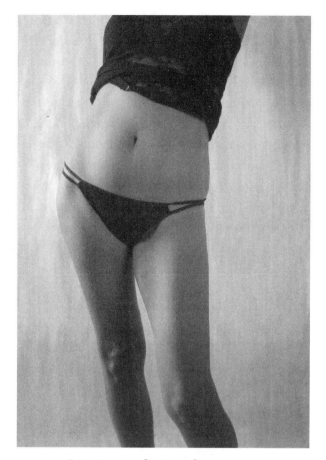

Scientia sexualis immediate sexiness

My professional work in the realm of relationships has convinced me of the limitations and failures of our "sexually liberated" scientia-sexualis culture as well as affirmed the benefits of applying the insights and practices of ars erotica. I have spent tens of thousands of hours using various ars erotica insights and practices to untangle complicated and embittered relationships—including blended-family and cross-cultural coparenting situations; ambivalent tensions regarding compatibility, marriage, and polyamory; and endlessly reverberating arguments on money, power struggles, communication issues, affairs, substance addictions, domestic violence, grief and depression, suicidal and psychotic episodes, the impacts of living with HIV, and in-law and traumatic childhood issues.

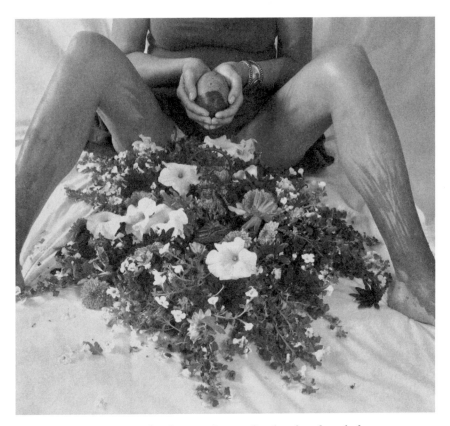

Ars erotica profundity combining fertility-lust-love-holiness

As a yoga mentor since 1974, copresident of the Association for Transpersonal Psychology since 1998, and director of the first "spiritual emergence service" in the world, the Kundalini Clinic (founded by Lee Sannella, M.D.) since 1984, I have also guided thousands of people worldwide in the unsettling experiences of kundalini awakening and urdhvaretas maturation. Questioning the past-oriented, scientia sexualis therapies of Freud, et al.,* I looked to yoga from the beginning of my career. Nearly forty years ago, I received the first federal grant to bring healing yoga and kirtan† to locked-up juveniles, as well as receiving other

---

*For my complete critique, see my book *Words from the Soul: Time, East-West Spirituality and Psychotherapeutic Narrative.*

†*Kirtan* is call-and-response chanting performed in India's *bhakti* devotional traditions.

first-ever grants to provide yoga-based help for the halfway-housed mentally ill. Indeed, many of the social and clinical problems that I have been arduously handling one by one for decades now seem resolvable or even preventable en masse, if only we were to live within a mature ars erotica culture.

As an instructor and twenty-year trustee for the California Institute of Integral Studies, the first East-West Spirituality graduate school in the United States, I oversaw training programs for thousands of "spiritually oriented" marriage and family therapists and co-created my own government-approved Sovatsky Method Couples Counseling trainings in Russia. I presented on *grihastha* (the stage of life devoted to marriage and family) in Indian colleges, including the University of Pune, to attune students to their own traditions of Divine Mother (ironically, this was just as Freudian Indologists were psychoanalyzing them away). I went on to lead retreats on urdhvaretas yoga and to give trainings on grihastha and *pariyanga* (boudoir yoga), in Europe, India, and South Africa, where I also led chanting gatherings with *sangoma* African shamans experienced with kundalini-type energies. In 2004 I helped produce *Awe to Action,* a conference-scale celebratory critique of the Burning Man Festival, and in 2008 I initiated a forty-country world conference in India supported by the office of the Dalai Lama with the goal of deepening the West's understanding of yoga and deepening bonds within the "world family."

Now, toward the end of my clinical career, I have reached new conclusions about the importance of yoga's ars erotica path and wanted to share these new insights by updating the first and second editions of this book. Entitled *Passions of Innocence* (1994) and *Eros, Consciousness, and Kundalini* (1999), those editions focused on the little-known ars erotica foundation of all Indian yoga known as *brahmacharya,* the "sublimative tantric celibacy" practice that is so different from the scientia sexualis priesthood celibacy of the Catholic Church.

This third and greatly expanded edition, retitled *Advanced Spiritual Intimacy,* focuses more on how yoga practices, reenvisioned as ars erotica, can enrich marital intimacies and support lifelong marriages. I have also expanded my guidance regarding the charismatic-energized yogic intimacy with God and the cosmos: kundalini awakening. *Advanced Spiritual Intimacy* is a journey from our current scientia sexualis world into the ars erotica of hatha yoga, the naturally creative lifelong marriage of grihastha, the conjugal all-puberties eroticism of pariyanga, and the inner marriage union within the body-mind-heart of yogis of all times.

The book also extends the incisive cultural critiques of Michel Foucault, Herbert Marcuse, Adam Curtis, and others regarding our unsustainable, desires-gone-rampant, family-broken modern world. We are living in a "global warming" of human bodies and romantic relationships brought forth by the well-meaning Freudian-Reichian-Burning Man overcorrections to the church's body-negating teachings.

These critiques are essential to free us from the negative impacts of both the moralistic scientia of Western religions and limited liberational scientia sexualis. This negativity started with biblical claims of an innate enmity between men and women, that the conception of new life is "the original sin" with maternal labor being a punishment for a primordial "fall from grace" and fleshy pleasures depicted as a slippery path to hell. Then, as a way out of that path to hell, came the popularization of psychoanalysis's bizarre map of fundamental Oedipal child-parent sexual longings and accompanying murderous animosities and a "sex drive" that the "institution" [sic] of lifelong marriage compromises.

Following this, a cavernous realm of "what's love got to do with it?" cyber porn was created alongside campaigns for less objectification of women and growing liberal concerns regarding a "porn problem,"* all happening within a mix of those decrying the looseness of promiscuity and others railing against legalizing gay marriage. Add to this tormented soup a psychoanalytically defined "sex drive" that has fourteen-year-olds "hooking up, because oral sex isn't really sex," an unswerving "drive" that must cut itself off contraceptively from the fertile seed powers (the Foucaultian *elixirs of life*) in order to be

---

*See Cindy Gallop's "Make Love Not Porn" TED Talk (http://blog.ted.com/2009 /12/02/cindy_gallop_ma), one of the "most talked about presentations" at the 2009 TED conference, on the negative effects of hardcore porn having become a main source of male sexual "education."

"orgasmically healthy," a theory proposed by Wilhelm Reich in his biophysics of human love.

Looking at our modern state of advertising, entertainment, and social media, it seems that we have now placed the entirety of human psychosexual maturation and lovemaking practices on the foundation of the puberty of the teen years. It's no wonder that a twenty-two-year-old Monica Lewinski was able to nearly topple the most powerful leader in the world via a series of adolescent-like hookups.

In contrast, yoga's ars erotica offers a lifelong path of urdhvaretas maturation, in which the seed-infused eroticism of pariyanga tantra and creative grihastha lifelong marriage and family life unfolds for all of us to enjoy and pass on to our children and they to theirs and they to theirs, ad infinitum. A simple yogic lifestyle nurtures the natural development of such maturity when no church or sex-liberation scientia is there to distract the teenager and young adult, as was the case in precolonial India for millennia.

Just as the global map of the earth radically transformed the preceding flat-earth maps of yore, the yogic urdhvaretas globe describes the possibilities of identity-and-pleasure-expanding development far more physical and throbbing than Freud's flat-earth, closed-dynamics idea of sublimated "idealizations" and more fully mature than his "final stage of the genital primacy ego," always struggling with its problematic superego and with family members and others. We have twelve-cylinder engines but have directions for only two or three, so we sputter along, breaking down over and over. This, we have been told by ego psychology, is "life."

Beyond the edge of the scientia sexualis map, the tantric ars erotica describes maturity (consisting of what can be understood as a transformative continuation of the teen puberty) as involving the entire cerebrospinal core and endocrine system, from perineum to pineal gland, which is capable of the "oceanic feelings" of love and oneness that Freud criticized as mere womb-regressive delusions but that the ars eroticas see as the most matured enlightenment of consciousness itself. Indeed, when the whole body is moved by these spinal awakenings, the *asanas* (positions) and *mudras* (gestures) of yoga become urdhvaretic—seed-infused tumescences of the Great Mother Kundalini that have barely anything in common with scientia sexuality or its repression or sublimation. We enter a whole new world.*

Nascent signs of these deeper retas (seed potentials) ripple throughout the charismatic ("being physically *moved*") spiritual traditions of all times, worldwide:

- Shaking of Shakers
- Quivering of Eastern Orthodox hesychasts
- "I got the Holy Ghost" shaking in Pentacostal and gospel congregations
- The throb of all-night, nature-entranced shamanic, African sangoma, *thxiasi num* awakened energies of the Bushman, South American Vodou trance dancers, and ancient Greek Dionysian revelers
- Esoterically undulating Middle Eastern belly dancers
- Inspired spinal-rocking Judaic davening and Sufi Islamic *zikr*
- *Uju kaya,* "ars erotically, blissfully tumescent spine" hidden in all still-sitting meditative paths, such as Buddhism, Jainism, Sikhism, and all contemplative Judeo-Christian traditions
- The ars eroto-yogic paths of pariyanga tantra
- The urdhvaretas-inspired *sahaja* or "spontaneously tumescent" performance of asanas that live quite outside of the standard yoga-studio scene of guided positions

Also noteworthy here are the 1950s gyrations of Elvis (the Pelvis) Presley, seeming like "purely musical-dance gestures," but genitally centered (and in public!), which initiated sixty years of youth-centric rock-and-roll world culture. Indeed, consider the now common,

---

*Interestingly, European discovery of India's spice and silk treasures was catalytic to shifting India's then-predominant wealth to struggling medieval European coffers and to the massive Eurocentric colonialist search for quicker sailing routes that helped reveal this global Earth. As irony would have it, it was Indian sailors who taught Columbus et al. the navigational methods they used to sail to (and typically exploit) numerous ars erotica cultures worldwide for hundreds of years.

crotch-grab dance "move." Concurrently, Afro-American rhythm-and-blues "soul music" carried the gospel vibes from their purely spiritual contexts into the then-developing cultural exuberance of scientia sexualis, with no little controversy and much loss of Holy Ghost-charismatic powers. Likewise, Westernized belly dancing lost its ars erotica core and became merely a scientia sexualis entertainment.

The vibratory energetics of uju kaya were often translated and (literally) sculpted out of Buddhism and other still-sitting paths, as they became formalized. For example, stone-sculpted yogis with ithyphallic penises were seen by European missionaries through their moralistic eyes as lustfully blasphemous and were commonly defaced, as were nipple-engorged breasts of goddess sculptures. How ironic that these ars erotically celibate or deified tumescences were misunderstood by the scientia missionary priests and even many modern (scientia-embedded) art scholars. (See the work of Thomas McEvilley for more on Western bowdlerizations of tantric and Buddhist art.)

Of all traditions, Indian Shiva-Shakti paths of urdhvaretas yoga have traced the unfoldment of charismatic (literally, "gifts from the divine") bodily awakenings in the most exquisite detail, which can be summarized as four main types of physical-spiritual maturation:

- The first type of unfoldment is that effected by practices involving the perineum and spine, in the form of both kundalini awakening and the more controlled, upright-sitting, spinal-energy-flowing meditation, which is found in Buddhism and other contemplative paths.
- Second is the path of the heart, grihastha: lifelong, compassionate, devotional, unbreakable marital-romantic and whole-lineage familial love, wherein procreation (and adoption) uplifts each human pair to godlike awe regarding the inherent meaningfulness of creating and caring for life itself.
- The third, pariyanga, is that of fully matured, "naturally entheogenic"* and pineal-orgasmic, conjugal eroticism (most

*Entheogen (literally, "generating the divine within") is the more spiritually attuned name for consciousness-enhancing chemistries such as LSD or psilocybin.

of which has not yet entered the popularized neo-tantra*).

- The ultimate *divya sharira,* "divine, whole-body, inner marriage puberty" maturation arises from *nirbija* (*nir,* fully exhausted or heatedly up-grown; *bija,* seed, a synonym for retas) *samadhi* (all-attention-spellbound-at-the-Source), also known as *nibbana* or *nirvana.* In India the resulting supremely happy inner marriage (with or without a partner) has been the sine qua non criterion for fully matured enlightenment for at least five thousand years. We see it manifested in whole-world-loving saints such as Buddha, Christ, Rumi, St. Francis, Teresa d'Avila, Adi Shankara, Amma-ji, Aurobindo and the Mother, Meher Baba, the Dalai Lama, and millions of others. Without such manifested maturity, no claims of enlightenment have ever been made in that ars erotica–steeped culture.

Within the ever maturing glandular chemistries and capacities of urdhvaretas, lovemaking emerges from a "perineum to pineal" neuroendocrine maturity of natural entheogens, our own urdhvaretas-matured secretions: versions of melatonin-serotonin-oxytocin-dimethyltryptamine-endorphin-semen-ova-androgen-estrogen-FSH-estrogen-testosterone-pheromones-vasopressin-dopamine-norepinephrine-ptyalin-lachrymose-erythrocytes and more.

Where does the maturing and consciousness-expanding power come from that can transform our bodily "elixir chemistries" (glandular *rasas,* "mood-essences") into inner "foods of the gods" (entheogens)? From untapped maturational potentials within the *siddhi*-seed-fertilities of life itself.[†] Why "untapped?" Because moralistic religions failed to fully explore their own charismatic sects and the massive scientia sexualis told

---

*According to Robert Thurman of Columbia University, only some 5 percent of the Indo-Tibetan archive has so far been translated and, I would add, typically without personal experience of the retas phenomena that is "lost in translation."

†Indeed, the ancient lore known as *rasa-yana* has always included ethically guarded "sacred botanicals" such as *Amanita muscaria* and *ephedra,* as in the Rig Vedic era communal rituals and other laboriously prepared precious mineral and plant "elixirs of immortality."

us their truths were "final" and only needed amplification via repetitive expert claims and endless media messaging. Indeed, many mature and less-than-mature ars erotica visiting gurus since the 1960s were swept away into the "anything-goes" mega-currents of scientia sexualis culture or their ars erotica teachings were misconstrued within the scientia spell. Those who weren't swept away show the way: a merging of lust-love-consciousness-reverence-fertility that also transforms each of these five terms from current scientia sexualis understandings to ars erotica embodied maturity.* Thus, too, the term, "tantric sex," like "ars erotica scientia sexualis," is a perfect oxymoron.

For example, all "semen-retention" neo-tantra practices should be considered as no more than learning-stage, mechanistic techniques within scientia sexualis–trapped bodies, while whole-spine-matured urdh-varetas bodies can entheogenize seed-related chemistries toward endless ecstasies, siddhis, lifelong loyalties, and *lila* (endless erotic play) far beyond the joyful or to-be-avoided "point of no return." And likewise, all contraceptives that make sex "safe from pregnancy" should be seen as no more than compromising training wheels en route to these same realms of wildly devotional love and lifelong, ever new explorations.

While every moment of yoga or meditation practice is a deeper step into urdhvaretas, in our current stage in the East-West cultural transmission this progress can be immediately neutralized by the gargantuan power of one hundred years and hundreds of trillions of dollars of scientia sexualis cultural momentum. "Liberated" nude yoga classes, for example, have less than nothing in common with—are in fact the exact *opposite* of—the clothingless ars erotica liberations of *naga* yogi ascetics of all times.

I have written *Advanced Spiritual Intimacy* to guide your traverse from the scientia sexualis and its global warming of bodies, souls, relationships, and families to the depths of ars erotica sustainable erotic ecology of urdhvaretas. As the Indic "Song of God" personified the ars

---

*All five—lust-love-consciousness-reverence-fertility—are implicitly merged and transformed in the untranslatable Sanskrit terms, *bindu, lingam,* and *yoni,* nearest cognates, respectively, for the medical terms, *semen, penis,* and *vagina,* and even slang terms like *cum, cock,* and *pussy.*

erotica: "I am that passion (*kama,* longing-desire) in beings that is in harmony with the eternal cosmos and leads to the complete maturation of each."[2]

In chapter 1, "Everything Will Change," I tell the story of my yogic awakening forty years ago, "when yoga was fab." Then, in chapter 2, "Entering the Mystery," I trace a path from today's scientia demystifications and despiritualized cynicism back to our original openness, curiosity, and innocence, and then to spiritual intimacies that are ars erotically matured and afire with the melted-together love-lust-fertility-profundity entheogenic elixirs.

Chapter 3, "Shared-Gender Mystery," reveals the reverberating "ecology of shared-gender mysteries" outside the current tumult of the scientia sexualis of commodified selves and too-oppositional "Mars-Venus" gender differences. In chapter 4, "Purposeful Urdhvaretas," I review some reasons people take up couples or solo urdhvaretas lifestyles for a time.

Chapter 5, "Yogic Anatomy and Transformation of the Ars Erotica Body," presents the seven *chakras,* the nonphysical energy centers that regulate the physical and the more subtle bodies, each with its own tonalities of passion. In chapter 6, "Commitment and Marriage as Grihastha Mysteries," the exploration of the lifelong retas mystery of couples and families focuses on the ars erotica commitment that is the very nature of human relationships as well as on the mystery of hidden potential and veiled union. The natural wonder and awe we feel when we approach the mystery of procreation is invoked in chapter 7, "The Passions and Mysteries of Fertility," particularly in the included meditation, "Retas Mysteries," which unlocks numerous yogic secrets as it guides you from conception through gestation and birth. The chapter also includes a section on the ars erotica "facts of life" for teenagers.

Chapter 8, "Within the Intimus," opens sixty-four of the many consciousness spaces of erotic-romantic sharing in which intimacy deepens and ars erotica awakenings can flourish. Then chapter 9, "Communication Yoga," offers twenty-one verbal asanas of creative communication and problem solving for couples.

Chapter 10, "Relational Worship," describes ars erotica practices that nurture the spinal puberties and lifelong love. In chapter 11, "Hatha Yoga as Ars Erotica," both individual and partnered ars erotica yoga practices are presented.

In chapter 12, "Sringara Rasa," the "Heaven Realm" of ars erotica, provides an alluring glimpse into naturally entheogenic conjugal eroticism. For those few who are "called," please know that the mystical solo brahmacharya urdhvaretas (the sine qua non of being an "advanced yogi") of chapter 13, "Brahmacharya," should be at least as esteemed for its ecstasies and wisdom as those of the "adults-only" conjugal pariyanga of chapter 12. Indeed, the legendary (and mostly scientia sexualis in its mentality) *Kama Sutra* "sex manual" closes with its own bow to brahmacharya.

As you journey with me you will discover that you already hold the "key" to these profound mysteries right where Mother left it at the base of your spine after she formed your body in utero. In fact, there are tiny charismatic keys moving within every cell of your body and major keys throbbing in your perineum, tingling in your genitals, longing in your love-creating heart, quivering under your taste-of-truth seeking tongue, and culminating in the center of your brain-mind, capable of entheogenizing consciousness—like a thousand-petaled lotus radiating ecstatic seed-keys everywhere!

1
Everything Will Change

*"Would you tell me, please, which way I ought to walk
from here?"*
"That depends a good deal on where you want to get to,"
said the Cat.

LEWIS CARROLL, ALICE IN WONDERLAND

A MOST UNUSUAL INVITATION

"Going *all* the way," said Rick, dropping the phrase casually into our conversation. His serenely rising pompadour, the confidence he so easily slipped into the word *all,* and especially his knowing glance let me know that, alas, at age thirteen, I was still a child and that my neighbor, at a towering sixteen, possessed secrets of incomparable power. Although I hadn't the slightest idea what he really meant (it was 1962), I knew enough not to admit it to anyone. Instead, I slinked away to where no one would see me, wrenched my belt buckle onto my left hip, and began Elvising an "I was *born* ready" pucker to some imaginary female audience. Five years later, after slipping out from a freshman college mixer with an equally enthralled coed, I found out what he meant.

On that lower bunk, while Sam the Sham roared on in the gym, veils were lifted and secrets disclosed. A new world of pleasures, precautions, and trepid anticipations surfaced, for I had (finally) gone "all the way." At least, that is what I thought, until another eight years later, when a most unexpected event occurred that suggested a realm of even greater hiddenness and secrecy. Suddenly the guiding star of sex that Rick, I, and everyone else I knew were following so devotedly shattered into a pulsing darkness, and "going all the way" began to stretch out before me endlessly.

I had been quietly relaxing at a weekend yoga retreat: healthy food, plenty of exercise, and time for reflection in a peaceful country setting. It was Sunday morning, and I was listening somewhat inattentively to our instructor's final talk on the ways of the mind and the needs of the heart and body: meditation, diet, self-acceptance—the usual topics for such an event. Suddenly the lecture took an unanticipated turn, and I thought I felt the room begin to sway:

Sigmund Freud was a very insightful psychologist. He saw very deeply into the sexual nature of man, but he did not see the whole picture. There are many stages of development beyond the teenager's puberty, but if you want to get to them you will have to go beyond his theories, therapies, and ways of "liberation." Are you ready to go on this yogic journey?

Beyond sex liberation? It was 1975, the time of free love, instant LSD enlightenments, the Age of Aquarius. Was this sparkling-eyed Indian yogi serious?

Not only was *he* serious, I too began to sense, as I had at age thirteen, that something mysterious and powerful was being revealed. And with that question, "Are you ready to go on this journey?" his provocative and fascinating words suddenly became a three-dimensional, outstretched hand that reached for my own. Should I take hold? It was only a lecture, wasn't it? I didn't have to *do* anything, did I?

Over the years I had heard scores of such talks, and I was always able to continue my life relatively unscathed. But this time I wondered if I would be walking away from something that, in Robert Frost's words, would make "all the difference." If this yogi was right, then was Western psychology wrong? If some "beyond sex" existed, why hadn't

I been told about it before? As these questions tugged and circled in my mind, one thing became alarmingly clear. I was actually considering stepping into a world of possibilities whose very existence I had never before suspected.

This step was something called urdhvaretas—a Sanskrit term meaning "a series of identity-maturing puberties, from perineum to pineal and beyond." And our confident teacher suggested we take a catalytic, "candle to candle," energetic transmission known as *shaktipat* that traced back two thousand years and "try it" by "marrying yoga, one-hundred percent" for a year and a quarter! "You mean *me*?" I gulped to myself, as a second barrage of feelings whirled through me: disbelief, challenge, fear, a solemn profundity, and then a deeply mysterious churning at the roots of my being, as if unawakened depths of my own body were being aroused and were also telling me, "We thought you'd never ask! *Here,* feel *this,* and *this* and *this,* see—there really is *more and more and more* . . ."

AWAKENING
DORMANT SEED POTENTIALS

The first six months of this totally monogamous, ars erotica marriage to yoga practices were intense. Several times while driving, my spinal sensations were so great that I had to pull over and let them subside. I would sing simple mantras and break into tears of "homecoming" to my own heart. My daily yoga practice was stirred into action by the first glimmers of the predawn rising sun, as pervasive yearnings animated bodily stretches into familiar and unfamiliar yoga asanas that now poured out of my outreaching arms, circling wrists, gesturing fingers, arching neck, swaying spine, dance-stepping legs and toes—catlike, gracefully, playfully, with outbursts of laughter or ferocious roaring—as I moved from one posture into the next and the next. In some innately intelligent way the shaktipat-catalyzed urdhvaretas was projecting my entire romantic-erotic nature into this marrying of yoga that seemed to be "liberating" my body and mind from the scientia sexualis "grip" of modern sexuality and redistributing and universalizing my "libido" throughout my body, making yoga, chanting, and meditation into my "one and only," most intimate lover.

My testes and perineum tingled like an infinity of scintillating star-flecks vibrating within me, yet without any arousals, erotic images, or desires for sexual activity (even including the habitual teen-developed happy urge to masturbate, which just went away). My forehead throbbed like a hymen being pressed toward some mystical union and my tongue and throat quivered blissfully in wordless fullness whenever I relaxed and turned within (as they have continued to do for decades).

This lingual quivering began in a mysterious way. I was in a darkened movie theater in Atlantic City watching *All the President's Men*, a film about the Watergate break-in, when all of a sudden this strange quivering broke into me and I grew mildly dizzy. A few weeks later I learned at another yoga retreat that a yogi in India (whom I had never met but who would become my main yoga guide and guru) had, at that very time, a decades-long maturational breakthrough in his advanced version of this same tongue-quivering puberty, known in Sanskrit as *khechari mudra,* and went ecstatically breathless for over an hour. My whole collegiate premed-instilled scientific paradigm of proximate causality began to shake, and shakes still.

Impossibly, or so I had thought until then, the entire frothy allure of swingin' sixties freedoms exited stage left. In its place was an awakened wisdom that stretched back thousands of years and unlocked the meaning of all sorts of yogic practices followed by hundreds of millions of yogis, Buddhas, philosophers, and mystical saints, worldwide, and clearly centralized in the scriptures some of them had left behind. The vast ars erotica of yoga explains why the yoga and enlightenment scene that has since burgeoned forth to uplift millions of lives has also come to appear ever more limited to me and to a growing number of yoga teachers. Could that first wave of enthusiasts have been so far off the mark in their fitness-focused practice on the mat as well as off the mat, taking in only so much as their hip scientia culture could easily assimilate? When I asked the publisher of *Yoga Journal* about my concerns, he said, "We are promoting a holistic lifestyle to as many people as possible, not some Indian, authentic yoga." Truth said.*

In fact there are yogas with a deeper inner heat than the hottest "hot room yoga," and intimate modes of attention more powerful than simply "being really present." Yoga has always been a path to eternal values and freedoms beyond the latest fashions and touted teachers. Maturity in lifelong married life, with a partner, or in the mystic wholeness of inner marriage, has been the gold standard and essential meaning of *hatha yoga*—"to yoke, to unite the sun (*ha*) and moon (*tha*) within—for tens of millions of yogis for thousands of years. There are soul-seed-powers more fecund with creativity than the popularized "Ultimate Power of Now," such as the "Father-activated, Kundalini Mother Power of lifelong maturation," or the deepest seed-activated "Till death do us part Love Passions, and you'll have to pry us apart, even then!"

And there are even more profound maturations whereby thousands of wise, charismatic, and loving Gandhis, Dalai Lamas, Buddhas, and hugging Mother Amma-jis might emerge from among today's eighteen million yogis to uplift our overly materialist, vengeance-riddled, and earth-pillaging cultures into a world of one caring and sustainable family—if only they knew the way. Such a vision inspired Buddhist writer Robert Thurman to seek grants for an ivy-league-level professional school, the Second Renaissance Institute, where meditation and other spiritual practices would prepare such leaders.

For me yogic marriage made humanitarian service the purpose of work and the neediest of the world my closest family. With a degree in religion from Princeton earned during the heights of peace demonstrations and campus consciousness expansion (I marched on Washington, went to Woodstock, and was voted the "Tim Leary" of my class), I went on to spend the next forty years bringing grihastha family counseling and yoga to impoverished schools, locked-up kids, broken shack-homes, seedy Atlantic City flophouses where the homeless mentally ill just

---

*In October 2013, Lululemon (yoga accessories mega-manufacturer) began marketing carrying bags on the theme of "moderation" with the word *brahmacharya* spelled out in a patchwork of candy, chocolates, French fries, and condoms (!), disclaiming that they aren't really experts in yoga. Truth said, again.

wait, glazed over, and into long-unvisited and withering elders in back-woods "rest-homes." And in the years since 1980, I cofounded a $34M green development project; co-created the first electronics-driven kirtan band, Axis Mundi; have clinically directed a traditional counseling center; and have been bringing my own version of spiritually attuned counseling to thousands of marriage and family therapy clients and students in the United States, Europe, India, post-apartheid South Africa, and Russia.

You could say that I, like millions of others, had gotten unfamously "spiritual," fueled in my case by this deeper connection to the universal seed forces (retas) of humanity, the empowering Mother Kundalini, and the poignant, "one family" purposes of why we are here. All the while, I researched the yogic map of complete maturation and ways to show others the limitations of the scientia sexualis, the happy but myopic and confounding sexuality that is everywhere. Foucault's hope became mine, too:

> In a different economy of bodies and pleasures, people will no longer quite understand how the ruses of [scientia] sexuality, and the power that sustains its organization, were able to subject us to that austere monarchy of sex, so that we became dedicated to the endless task of forcing its secret, of exacting the truest confessions from its shadow . . . having us believe that our "liberation" is in the balance.[1]

In his reversed characterization of our modern era of "sexual liberation" as the "austere monarchy of sex," Foucault goads us toward somewhere else, outside this ironic, compelled "austerity," as I have tried to convey by writing in the *kavi* (poetic) yogic tradition, which you will find interspersed and page-centered throughout this book. Please read these verses, drink them, as guided meditations, in keeping with the path most famously employed by the ars erotica kavi-genius Rumi. Poetry tries to effect a transformation, like turning water into wine, in which ordinary words become "verse-wine," engendering permission to love beyond the norms, by opening the heart-space of "the endless wedding feast." (Sanskrit terms in the verses that are not defined in the text itself can all be found in the glossary).

Far beyond the thrall of the teenaged awakening
Nature has hidden in us
numerous rare and mysterious erotic reflexes
and transformative puberties
(except for kundalini, completely unknown to modern
        times—
did we really believe we had discovered
everything there is about the erotic universe?)
the fleshy basis of all spiritual yearning
that only an ever-deeper passion might awaken:
shuddering genital reversals vajroli mudra, shakti
        chalani,
that emerge in meditative depths
or only after the second hour of embrace,
spinal surges kundalini shakti, *davening,*
Quakering, Shakering, zikr-ing, holy ghosting,
involving spellbinding novitiates of seed-retas
        maturation,
excessively devotional surrenders
requiring an ease with tears
at the thought of it all,
and even more distant throat-choking pharyngeal
        hypoglossal arousals,
khechari mudra,
soaring into consummate pineal emissions
soma rasa, *nectar of the gods,*
inebriating the inmost soul
with breathless beauties everywhere,
completing itself perhaps a dozen lifetimes from now.
In a different economy of bodies and pleasures
we might call these awakenings "postgenital puberties"
as in this ancient name for Yoga: shamanica medhra,

"the going-beyond-genital-awakenings"
—but beyond into what?

As urdhvaretas maturity opened me over the decades to the realm of fully seed-infused erotic pariyanga or boudoir yoga, it was like heaven and earth combined, fueled by naturally entheogenic passions far beyond that "austere monarchy" of scientia sex:

> *Two people chained to one another in endless causality*
> *by their reverberating attractions to one another,*
> *endless irresistibility inciting endless irresistibility,*
> *chemical fusion reactions of the entire polarized*
>   *universe.*
> *Every glistening retas-permeated cell poised aimed at*
>   *him, at her,*
> *and nothing else is what every living gendered fiber*
>   *wants,*
> *has ever wanted,*
> *a hundred a thousand a million years.*

After fifty-two years I have come to believe that I have seen and gone "all the way" to erotic places Rick and I never dreamed were possible back in the hot-rod and belt-buckle era of 1962, "when we was fab."

URDHVARETAS FIRST BURSTS
IN THE MODERN WEST

The current studio yoga and "Now" enlightenment scene is like merely putting a toe into the sandy shores of the further-out, oceanic depths of the Eastern truths of the body and consciousness accessed through an urdhvaretas "marriage to yoga, one-hundred percent." Consider the description given by the modern-era Indian yogi and author of *Kundalini, The Evolutionary Energy in Man*, Gopi Krishna, of his own perineum-to-pineal urdhvaretas awakening of Mother Kundalini. He had merely turned the right keys and "mushroomed" (without substances) into what yoga calls the *anandamaya-kosha,* "quantum-causal-bliss-body" (see chapter 5 on yogic ars erotica anatomy), which I call one of the many "rooms" or "inner spaces" of the *intimus,* the most interior, (in chapter 8):

> Suddenly, with a roar like that of a waterfall, I felt a stream of liquid light entering my brain through the spinal cord. . . . The illumination grew brighter and brighter, the roaring louder, I experienced a rocking sensation and then felt myself slipping out of my body, entirely enveloped in a halo of light. . . . It grew wider and wider, spreading outward while the body, normally the immediate object of its perception, appeared to have receded into the distance until I became entirely unconscious of it. I was now all consciousness without any outline, without any idea of corporeal appendage, without any feeling or sensation coming from the senses, immersed in a sea of light simultaneously conscious and aware at every point, spread out, as it were, in all directions without any barrier or material obstruction. I was no longer myself, or to be more accurate, no longer as I knew myself to be . . . but instead was a vast circle of consciousness in which the body was but a point, bathed in light and in a state of exultation and happiness impossible to describe.[2]

Krishna's many books captured the attention of scientia-trained clinicians such as my predecessor, Lee Sannella, M.D., cofounder of the first "spiritual emergence" service, the Kundalini Clinic, and author of the 1977 meme-setting book, *Kundalini: Psychosis or Transcendence?* which helped other transpersonal colleagues to modify the American Psychiatric Association's bible, the *DSM-IV.** Sannella's book opens by comparing kundalini awakening with the often difficult but profoundly meaningful seed-force throes of childbirth. Indeed, the Cross-cultural

---

*See my *Words from the Soul* and "Clinical Forms of Love Inspired by Meher Baba's Mast Work" on the distinctions between sought-after "meditative states" and the *Diagnostic and Statistical Manual of Mental Disorders* (*DSM*'s) "Depersonalization Disorder" and also on the underappreciated challenges that emerge during extremely positive spiritual experiences that were unmentioned in *DSM* v.62.89 "Religious Issues" section.

Disorders section of the *DSM-IV* lists a variety of seed concerns as being noteworthy for many Asian cultures but ends there.

Likewise, in complete congruence with the frothy scientia sexualis sixties and since, Krishna's emphatic inclusion of the essential role of the retas seed forces in kundalini processes "to feed the inner man" has been continuously ignored. Thus, today, many in our scientia sexualis culture talk of and teach about their "kundalini awakenings" or their "ultimate Now awakenings," but do not include or live in the urdhvare-tas mystery. Scientia sexualis has indeed reigned as an austere monarchy, ignoring centermost profundities within the ars eroticas of other cultures and simultaneously blinding itself to even its most liberal critics.

For example, as early as 1932 and without much of an alternative in mind, psychedelic initiate and humanistic spiritualist, Aldous Huxley wondered if the nascent scientia sexualis liberation might be a premonition of a darkly fraught "brave new world" of easily accessible sexual liaisons and eugenically efficient reproduction that masked a perditious narrowing of human warmth and intimacy.

Likewise, Marxist philosopher Herbert Marcuse saw the scientia sexualis as a "repressive de-sublimation" of eros into a mushrooming of "desire" that fueled an unsustainably rapacious capitalism, a hypothesis explored in the cogent BBC four-hour documentary, *The Century of the Self,* on the creation of advertising "spin" by Freud's nephew, Edward Bernays.

"Spin" has proven to be the most insidious exploitation of natural bodily arousals since the Jesuit Inquisition, not as a "repression of wayward passions," but as an exploitative despiritualization of love and beauty itself in order to (like a hip drug dealer) sell more of what we are told we "gotta have!" For "it's not how long you make it, it's how you make it long" (the double-entendre advertising spin used to launch Winston's long cigarettes*). Marcuse's proffered response in *Eros*

---

*This ad (http://blog.modernmechanix.com/its-not-how-long-you-make-it) appeared amid the outreach of the producers of these carcinogenic products in ever more gender-competitive ways such as Marlborough Men and Virginia Slims and "get 'em addicted at first glimmer of puberty," cartoonish Joe, the "phallic-cephalic" camel (in an ad that was eventually banished, http://adstrategy.wordpress.com/2010/11/17/joe-camel).

and Civilization in 1955, though vague, was a "spiritualization of the instincts."

Even Marty Klein, past president of the Society for the Scientific Study of Sexuality and a chief architect of the scientia sexualis for forty years, has recently written in *Sexual Intelligence* that the narratives, theories, and stories we create about sex are more powerful than "sex" itself in determining how "sexuality" unfolds in people's lives—not the mere freeing up of an unswerving "sex-desire." Freud, who excommunicated Jung from the psychoanalytic fold for putting "sexual energy" into a spiritual context, would be rolling over in his grave to read Dr. Klein's blasphemy.

As a first step toward the ars erotica, hipper sectors of the scientia sexualis now speak of "the spirituality of sacred sex." The prolonged, nonejaculatory, and passionate "fucking one's partner to God" of field leader David Deida counters Reich's centralized "function of the orgasm" with an endless *karezza* sexuality for men and multiple, deep orgasms (not shallow "monkey orgasms," as Deida quips) for women. Rajneesh-Osho's teaching "that brahmacharya is diamond and sex is coal" was eschewed, leaving him with the also true reputation of being the "sex guru." Thus, too, Pulitzer winner and *New York Times* science page journalist William Broad, chose "thinking-off" (touchless fantasy masturbation) as his hint-of-a-step toward the "deeper" aspects of yoga and tantra in his scientia yoga book, *The Science of Yoga,* which was featured on the front page of the *Times.*

In contrast, the following are full steps forward in the shift from monarchical scientia sexualis (including the neo-tantras) to ars erotica terra firma:

- Recentering with "retas entheogenic profundity" where "sex-desire pleasures" once reigned supreme, for without the retas seeds potencies of all life that are the gold standard of five thousand years of Indian ars erotica explorations, the neo-teachings, however beneficial, are not backed by this time-honored "gold"
- Exploring where, and in what moods, partners might focus their attentions upon genitals, mouths, anuses, perineums, feet, ears,

eyes, lips, tongues, breasts, feeling-hearts, and the glowing inner-self of one another

- Revaluing "happy-ending," simply disposable "cum," vaginal "lubrication," and all other "sex-fertility-love-bonding hormones" as the hermetically prized, alchemically matured, male and female *elixirs of life* itself: entheogenic retas (seed energies), *ojas* (radiance), *auras* (golden glow), *madhu* (intoxicating honey-mead), *virya* (virility virtue), *amrita* (immortality-ambrosia essence), and *soma rasa* (deity-ambrosia essence)

- Discovering how these and other matured essences become the hormonal/energetic basis that unites lifelong, creative love-lust-fertility-profundity-maturity into a singular and transformative potency

- Learning how the male "retention" included in pop neo-tantra "training wheels" becomes endless erotic worship within the far more expansive and matured entheogenic bodies of ars erotica partners

- Embracing a "new" vocabulary (provided by Sanskrit) to name the then-occurring sensations, such as: shakti chalani (moving the divine feminine), *brahmacharya urdhvaretas* (up-blossoming inner marriage seed energies), *shambhavi mudra* (tumescently ecstatic eyes in divine-light-seeing delight ocular gesture), khechari mudra (tumescent-tongue evoking the pineal nectared orgasm), and pari-yanga (khechari mudra–based endless worship lovemaking)

- Seeing how the spine, forehead, throat, and pineal become primary realms of erotic rapport and arousal, not as scientia arousals of desire, but within the ars erotica's "new economy of bodies"

- Reclaiming the profundity and natural ease of lifelong, creative marriage and family life, far beyond today's liberalized divorce accommodations and the ever-haunting ghost of Adam and Eve's primordial marital enmity and "flesh-fallen" beliefs about erotic attraction, child conception, and worldly life

Based in overarching historical and linguistic analyses, language philosopher Ludwig Wittgenstein noted how theories create self-enclosed "forms of life, language-behavior games," Martin Heidegger lyricized how language itself "conceals, as it reveals," and Thomas Kuhn's paradigm analysis showed how dominant theories ignore and even squelch any contradictory information. The fact that conservatives and liberals cannot even agree on when respect for life processes should begin or what "natural" adult love is or is not shows the self-persuasive power of one's ideological paradigm or "group language-game."

Thus, consider the complete transitioning from our current desire-centric scientia sexualis world into an ars erotica world. In such an ars erotically liberated culture, all the elements of "eros" would change. For example, the current Internet space occupied by a mega-industry of cyberpornography would instead be filled with spellbinding ars erotica websites because, as Foucault would note, "profundity" feels better than endlessly repetitive and more extreme cyberporn permutations of (de-seeded) sex-desire (not because it is "morally superior"). There would be other changes too, such as in flirtation and dating, gender identifications, child conception, love songs and musical energizations, lifelong marriage, asana instruction, enlightenment, the treatment of charismatics, and the exploration of currently discarded monastic developmental esoterica underlying all universities. The value of "normative" sexological statistics and the chronic conservative vs. liberal sexo-moral debates would all also change. Indeed, "everything" would change.

Such radical cultural changes represent the dramatic power of a "techno-paradigm shift"—like the mere forty-year shift from typewriters, written/mailed letters, and libraries to laptops, e-mail, and Google. Just as the LSD serotonin rush of consciousness-truth threatened the popularity of feel-good alcohol in the sixties, entheogenic ars eroticism will test the simpler, de-seeded testosterone and estrogen allure of sex-desire.

In such a context, urdhvaretas converts will then roll their eyes and, as Foucault put it, "no longer quite understand how the ruses of [scientia] sexuality, and the power that sustains its organization, were able to subject us to that austere monarchy of [scientia] sex" for so long. Perhaps another glimpse into pariyanga will explain and allure:

With the secret spinal passageway spiraling upward
you could ambrosially lap and hungrily devour all
    the way up to my mind
so your perfect feathery lips were now in my mind
licking the interior darkness billowing responsively in
    being licked,
my mind licking back, leaving wet radiances on your
    lips,
carefully reaching into the billowing Infinity

Your back purrs should I even glance at its central
    groove
arising hidden and dark from the violet-tinged
    perineal trikonam
cresting up and smoothly down into the sacral well
reaching forward between your praying
    shoulder-blades
then burying into your softest neck flesh beneath the
    wisps of child hairs
diving into brainstem where seething rhythms of the
    sapient universe
flare invisibly a milky-starry conflagration of
    electrified axons dendrites
filled with tigers' movements, panthers' eyes,
a million million combinations
to trigger throbbing hips upstretched hands hearts
    lips

Who was I who you? For those hours,
it no longer mattered who was who,
loving each other's hungers as one's own.
I looked out my eyes and was you, but you floating
    in us.
Happy feeling how beautiful you are from the inside,
become those silky shoulders I love to caress,

that smile now mine,
not the slightest worry of losing my way back,
what difference would it really make?
We would as well be each other as ourselves,
so in love in awe of each other were we.

If the modern yoga and neo-tantra of the current eighteen million enthusiasts is reunderstood as seed-infused ars erotica, with a few
dozen senior urdhvaretas master teachers giving profound shaktipat
energetic initiations to a few hundred thousand of them, a massive
paradigm shift will shake and quake and holy-ghost throughout the
entire scene of studio yoga and nearly bodiless "Enlightenment Now"
pop spirituality.

REENVISIONING FAMILY LIFE

It was not until 2009, after nearly forty years of teaching that family
life is a kind of "melodrama" to test one's actual spiritual growth, that
Ram Dass, the coiner in 1970 of the "Be Here Now" galacto-meme,
awoke to a critical error in his teachings on soul love and familial
relationships. Via his DNA-verified paternity and grand-paternity and
family reunion, he "developed a deeper understanding of the love parents feel for their children and began to see that personal and soul
love are not mutually exclusive but can coexist in nourishing ways."[3]

In the ars erotica, family life is neither a Freudian-conflicted hot-
house nor a sidebar melodrama. It is the primordial retas seed mystery
naturally embodying, procreating, and nurturing life itself.

Within grihastha, family life is a day-to-day "urdhvaretic meditation on life itself" of lovers or spouses beholding, delighting, and
arousing one another toward heart-and-soul adult puberties; facing
life issues, parenting conundrums, and paying bills together as help-
mates; parents musing about their gestating babies, beholding the
birth and daily maturation of their children and of the latter looking with love and respect upon their aging parents; and, decades
later, the meditation upon the marriages of one's children; and the

supernourishing glow of newborn grandchildren and perhaps mega-glow of great-grandchildren and the poignant caring for wizened elder parents, unto their often incontinent, gaunt, and overwhelming deaths by their now-adult and ever-aging "adult children," tracing forward and back in time, ad infinitum.

In this highly nourishing rasa-juicy ars erotica universe, lifelong creative marriage becomes the natural order of the sun-moon-stars universe, for the vast majority. The ars erotica universe gives humans more than most all of us need to create lifelong loves. Indian, Tibetan, and Navajo divorce rates of 1.1, 3.8, and 4.8 percent respectively speak of an ars erotica bonding that rarely breaks,* in contrast to U.S. and all major scientia sexualis cultures worldwide, with rates fluctuating between 40 and 50 percent over the past twenty years for first marriages and statistics of 60 percent for second and 70 percent for third marriages in the United States, and such high rates of nonmarried breakups that we normalize them as a lifestyle of "serial monogamy."[4] Even allowing for a tripling of the low divorce rates in ars erotica cultures to accommodate troubled, intact marriages, the rates are a fraction of the scientia sexualis cultural rates.[†]

> *In a different economy of bodies and pleasures*
> *each couple a universe unto themselves,*
> *sheltering their children, grand- and*
> *   great-grand-children*
> *in expanding overlapping bio-radiant fields of gender*
> *   worship,*
> *all growing magnificently in love and awe.*
> *Ten-thousand couples become a* sangha *(community),*
> *ten-thousand sanghas a* pradesh *(state),*

---

*For better or worse, those rates have begun to rise as scientia sexualis spreads.
†For a comprehensive, nonideological study of the lifelong, destructive effects of contemporary American divorce, see Wallerstein, *The Unexpected Legacy of Divorce.* For research on positive effects of supportive counseling for families with young children, see the work of Carolyn Pape Cowan at the University of California, Berkeley: http://tinyurl.com/m7l27gy.

ten-thousand states a loka *(realm),*
ten realms the world, Vasudaiva kutumbakam—
"The world is, indeed, one family."
One billion vibrant planetary households,
sacred grihastha, the center that holds each and all
the lion with the lamb,
the endless wedding feast,
gender worship on high,
manifested on earth as it is in heaven.
Throw open the secret passage!

2
Entering the Mystery

Moving from Cynical Certainty
to Spiritual Intimacies

SOMETHING HIDDEN IS GOING ON

In 1985 I published a study of the sexual experiences and beliefs of people who saw themselves as sexually liberated or who were practicing neo-tantric or brahmacharya yogas. As I listened to my interviewees, I heard how each one was being allured by something hidden within her- or himself, within another, or within the greater universe. I concluded that drawing-closer-to-something-hidden is the essential erotic act, whether by means of conventional sex, neo-tantra, or brahmacharya yogas.

Thus, the concealing-while-revealing powers of the double entendre and the discreetly veiled gesture serve erotic intentions very well, for they all deftly convey that *something* hidden is going on. The sense of ambiguity inherent in such communications alluringly and undeniably signals that we are moving from nonerotic to more *intimate* domains. A tingle here, a spark there—from the suggestive smile of a lingering stranger whose eyes stir our secret hopes, to the Buddha's trace of a smile hinting at a spiritual bliss barely veiled by the play of worldly illusions.

The question "What exactly is this hiddenness?" led me more deeply toward the essence of eros—into the feeling of mystery itself. Sex feels hidden from us not because any authority or moral code has hidden it but because it *is*, intrinsically, archetypally, and ontologically, of the Hidden. For eros is not a "thing" but an essential quality-that-allures, which, like retas wisdom, *unfolds* with deepest DNA mysteries or even deeper than science has yet grasped. It is the secrecy within any secret, the hiddenness within anything veiled, the possibility of a sexual or talisman fetish in every object, and the Mystery within anything suggesting further revelations. From that magnetically suggestive glint in your parents', your grandparents', and their parents' and grandparents' eyes when each couple first met, to the retas fertility possibilities of your future grandchildren "inside" you and another being, alluring you to inevitably meet.

From endless tabloid exposés to the latest anatomical discoveries, we muse endlessly about eros, not merely because we are so liberated (or addicted), but because *suggestiveness* grips us, as if in a page-turning mystery, with always another page to turn: hemlines go up, then down, then up again, for the curtain must reveal and conceal. Interpretations can ever shift, too: a Freudian penis in every cigar and cosmic *lingam* (fertile awe-inspiring phallus) in every penis, a vagina in every Freudian concavity and a *yoni mudra* (nurturing womb source of all beings delight mind gesture) in every vagina-womb or in the meditative darkness when you close your eyes. The ambiguous "come-up-and-see-me-sometime" and "have-you-seen-my-etchings?" serve as covert invitations into the intimus, where the more intimate of rites might be revealed, including secret, two-thousand-year-old yogic energy transmissions of shaktipat that can open invisible channels in your perineum-to-pineal path to Shiva-Shakti inner bliss. Hiddenness, mysteries, and powers beyond "the mundane" peek out everywhere, too.

The redefinition of eros as mystery adds the living touch of mercurial and multilayered nuance to a sexual liberation that has been painted in broadly political strokes. Within this context of an ever-broadening mystery, a sexuality of great secrecy emerges—not because any person or dogma has repressively kept it away from us. The mystery grows deeper as we step out of the overly familiar grooves and conventions of current sexual knowledge. We don't know what we didn't know until *after* we have learned something new!

FIVE DEGREES OF APPROACH

There is always *more* to consider, even physical immortality, as was the central aim of all yogis some six hundred years ago, or a utopian world in which all live together in peaceful, one-creative-family rapport, perhaps the deepest longing of everyone now alive. As D. H. Lawrence noted in *The Plumed Serpent,* "How wonderful sex can be, when men keep it powerful and sacred, and it fills the world! Like sunshine through and through one!" To understand eros we may need to leave the realms of certainty to study everything we can about mystery, on its own terms.

Sit quietly with your eyes closed and feel the many pulsings in your body. Become aware of your most immediate erotic sensation; feel the sensation pulsate, shift, and move throughout some bodily locale. Go more deeply into the details of this feeling without doing anything about it.

As sexual-love fantasies come and go, sense one nuance or tonality of sensation arise, throb, stir, and pass in loins, penis, vagina, testicles, womb, ovaries, prostate, anus, legs, chest, gut, throat, eyes, fingertips, toes. Feel the warm rushes and their fleeting evaporations, the currents of excitement with their cresting heat and their withering falls, lighting up again in some other, deeper visceral dimension. This seething flow of feelings, when traced to its subtlest levels, is the elusive erotic seed mystery about which we articulate our numerous and divergent interpretations and opinions and from which we enact our manifold forms of love and pleasure.

From smitten allurement and well-meaning plans to reverential awe, and then to disappointments and cynical bitterness and back again, such are the meandering thoughts and passions that filter through the innocence of our awareness. In the next sections we will trace the hopes of erotic mystery from their too-common deteriorations into shared moods of cynicism and misanthropy to those throbbing with living hopefulness and creative power that allure with the possibilities of an ars erotica heaven-on-earth for all.

- The bitterly opinionated passion of *cynical certainties* nursed on personal resentments and the media's magnification of our culture's more lurid desperations and tragedies
- The more hopeful, temporarily useful but overgeneralized *demystified certainties* of sexological science, popular psychology, and traditional moralities that in strangely divergent ways try to guide us toward better or healthier habits of living
- The pulse-quickening and alluringly alive waters of *suggestive ambiguities,* which will always rock our demystified, pat certainties and crack even our most cynical rigidities with their siren calls of possibilities hidden betwixt and between more decisive erotic viewpoints or theories
- The profoundly shuddering and captivating flickers of *evanescent subtleties,* which make us feel quite awesomely that right *Now,* you and I are the inexplicable, living, aging, creating, and dying-away mystery itself
- The meditatively spellbinding hush of the innermost intimus, where eros-as-sheer-mystery unfurls in a shimmering sanctity and where the deepest energies of Mother Kundalini and urdhvaretas awaken entheogenic puberties in us, which, even in these times of yoga and "Now" enlightenments, lie both far ahead and exquisitely nearer than the nearest.

I have charted five degrees of approach to the urdhvaretas mystery in the figure on the following page. Each mood is guarded from the next by the dubious warning, "Beware! That next degree is too wondrous to be true!" This attitudinal gatekeeper of our wavering hopes and credulity must maintain certainty in our current erotic knowledge and skepticisms, for maintaining our orderly and familiar beliefs is her job. However, at the same time, she wonders; she knows better; she suspects there is more.

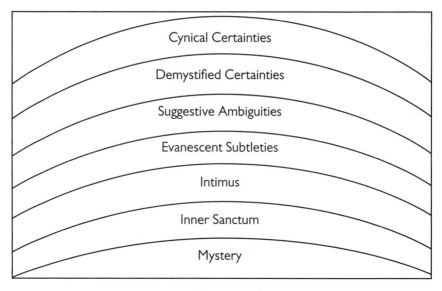

Entering the auras of mystery

So she opens the first gate, and we proceed. Then, having given up her grim outpost in cynicism and, after that, her persuasive, authoritative uniform of demystified certainty, she nakedly flings herself into suggestive erotic ambiguities, evanescent subtleties, and, finally, the wonders of mystery itself. The gatekeeper, we find, is our own focusable yet oft wavering ego-mind (endearingly called "the monkey-mind" in Buddhist literature). And our pathway to her erotic freedom? It is our willingness to believe in the ars erotica scriptures and our "yogic experiences," however distant and rare, more than in the reigning scientia sexualis that is everywhere.

Cynical Certainty

On the outer edges of eros, wounded, disillusioned, and estranged from perceiving our own innocence and that of others, is where we sometimes stand, having grown cold, bitterly so, and cynical in our too-certain pronouncements about the subtle warmth inside. Indeed, cynical certainty has become ubiquitous in our modern, post-*Father Knows Best*, and romantically broken culture, amplified in numerous "the darkest ways must be shown" *Fatal Attraction* type of movies, "it'll end in tears" type of songs, and horrific news stories that both reflect back and shape our knowledge of "life." With privately resentful grumblings or loudly strident sexo-political railings and counter-railings, the cynical ones scoff, "The real truth is on tabloid TV; it's all sex and power. And remember, the wages of sin are death!"

Regarding homosexuality, homophobia and internalized homophobia prevail. Intoxicatingly passionate, such cynical certainties can rule one's life for decades. In heterosexuality, misanthropy and misogyny have tango-danced themselves into a litigious-like frenzy of distrust and hopeless passivities or retaliations.

"There is no love! Just take what you want!" or "Just forget it all, go celibate!" "The fallen gurus and priests prove that any form of celibacy is an impossible pretense! Or maybe they just can't perform!" "Trust no one, for they'll use you every time!" Such are the pained, wounded, and soured pronouncements of cynical certainty.

But perhaps someday a curiosity arises; we read a self-help book, begin therapy, or take up yoga classes in a church basement. Perhaps a Bible is looked at or a liberating report is published, and our eyes are opened. We shed tears of remorse, and our lives turn toward more alluring radiances. Something "too good to be true" is glimmering as a "maybe so."

We come across the old wine of salvation-seeking in the new bottles of psychology: be more grateful, forgive more, slow down and smell the roses. Some titles do betray lingering cynicism—*Smart Women, Foolish Choices*—or overblown images of vast differences—*Men Are from Mars, Women Are from Venus*—but all these teachings mean well. With innocence renewed, we enter demystified certainties.

Demystified Certainty

Inside the portico it is a bit warmer. We feel more hopeful, willingly guided by an expert voice with clear definitions about good habits and exercises, the "good news." We learn of "natural drives," "four-phased orgasms," "scientifically verified differences (or similarities) between men and women." "Doing yoga," we hear, "is really good for you." "Family values are critical!" "Gay marriage must be legalized!"

We are inside the sociocultural system now, collectively rooting for our particular left, right, or mid-road sexo-political agenda. Regarding abortion, for example, liberals take to the streets, knowing it to be rightful and necessary, while conservatives form human barricades, convinced it is unquestionably evil. Regarding a more solitary matter, masturbation is celebrated by one group as a self-loving relaxation and shunned by the other as a wasteful vice. Porno is a fifth amendment right and exciting and healthy or it horrifically objectifies women and dehumanizes sex and should be heavily restricted or banned. Such demystifying certainties about everything erotic impassion and guide each adherent, as best as possible, given these demystified, constrictive circumstances.

Lists of discrete "emotional needs" are drawn up by the popularizing psychologists, and the healing way of the inner child is outlined in step-by-step fashion. All of the difficulties of erotic life seem to be easily explained by one morality or school of therapy or another or by the proper sociopolitical analysis. Insightful, compassionate, and encouraging, but still far too certain, these generalizations and formulaic approaches to eros refresh us but are overprocessed and deeply embedded in the binary limitations of scientia sexualis: right/wrong, or repression/expression, or sexual/spiritual, and so on. Yes, clarity and lists of "my feelings, my needs" can be temporarily helpful, but if we do not move on to the greater ars erotica mystery, the usefulness of these recovering, rehabilitative ways becomes stagnant.

Like the strict certainties of moral codes of an older vintage, such clarity can become well-intended help that binds. Becoming too confident, we can even find ourselves using pop formulas such as "All love is just an addiction; everyone is a codependent" against ourselves and others when they don't really apply.

As in the demystified certainty of the scientist, the partisaned conviction of the politico, and the coolness of the sexual sophisticate, an aloof confidence lets us know we have to go further than unambiguous generalizations to enter the living currents of erotic mystery. We must surrender more of our certainties and uncover the ever-shifting subatomics of the erotic matrix of suggestivity, evanescence, and the well-guarded intimus. Indeed, we are allured by the very mention of such things.

Suggestive Ambiguity

Suggestive ambiguities, given their greater proximity to the seed-infused mystery, are indeed far more powerful than demystified certainties of pop therapists, no matter how renowned. This class of ever-beckoning erotic communications includes double entendres, vocalized innuendos, veiled gestures, synchronous coincidences, and foreshadowing dreams. In their inherent ambiguity they imply and allure with suspense and excitement, but not without also radiating daring moods of uncertainty and trepidation.

The lecture hall is packed, with all eyes upon the gesturing figure at the podium who is expounding on the demystification of the ways of love. As the speaker's words, "mystified relationships cannot stand up to the natural pressures of reality" resound boldly, that strikingly attractive individual in the fourth row catches your eye and your heart begins to swell, and everything else fades away.

When he turns in your direction and your gazes meet in a stunning shyness and with quiet, eyes-dropping smiles, only the throb of a mystery stirred brims in your every cell. What does this mean? You imagine your first date with each other, lovemaking, moving in with each other (will we have the same tastes?), even the hair color of your children. Simultaneously, the lecturer's amplified words of demystified certainty drift high in the air: "Too often we engage in relationships based in some form of romantic fantasies. . . ." But you are only awaiting the break when you can go down to the fourth row.

During the break, you ignore all the lecturer said and approach him. Your first flirting question is a gift for both of you—it is a gift that you give yourself and a gift to him too: "I like your tie, where did you find such a tie?" He will thank you (for the gift of your courage and willingness to merely ask the first question and for complimenting his tie, and—and this is the most important part—for moving with him toward this fleeting, energized romantic space where two people can become special to one another, among the thousands of others).

As he answers you, he is making you special to him, in that moment. When he tells you where he bought it, you can go a little further into this seed power—infused space by making the compliment more personal by saying, "I like the way you answered my question, so direct (or with such humor, or with such surprise, or . . .).

It is not merely his verbal answer (the name of the store) that you can respond to, it is the way he responded that you should also notice. Now, you are really talking about him, his way of doing something: this is very personal. (Of course, cynicism can emerge in this ambiguity: "This is just a pickup line; what a slick player!" Or, "This line works on chicks, all the time!")

If you merely say, "I don't know that store, where is it?" then you are talking road maps and helping the store location to get well known. Who cares about that? Not you. If you say, "Oh, I also shop at that same store," this makes a little more connection. But if you watch and listen to him as he answers, you will have something to say about his very way of being. For example: "You know, your smile lit up when you told me the tie was a gift from your favorite aunt. I felt very happy for you and for your aunt that you could smile like that when you thought about her, even for a moment!" Now you are enjoying his life, his family, and projecting yourself into his aunt's "shoes" and letting him know that his love of his aunt is a wonderful thing. You are almost in his family by now!

If he gives you the compliment of saying back to you, "What a lovely thing to say about me and my aunt!" then you have a great partner who already knows the grihastha alchemical dance. If he continues, "I thoroughly enjoyed imagining my aunt seeing your smile," he will have added another powerful churn to the heart-opening rasas. And then you say, "You have an amazing imagination!" And he says, "Thank you for saying that; it makes me happy for you to appreciate my imagination! Can you guess what I am imagining now?" (Here the seed-energies of eroticism emerge within the veils of a not-so-simple question, and partners begin making tentative pledges within the creativity of two people believing in the "good intentions" of one another.)

And you say, "Not only can I imagine it, I am with you in it as well!" And he says, "The rest of the world has faded away. It is only you and me in this dream together that is Real." And you say, "This is a dream that I have been waiting to wake up into for my whole life." And he says, "Yes, *this is just the beginning!" With the lifelong developmental map of urdh-varetas to guide the two of you, the untapped, entheogenic powers of your intercatalyzing ways will make good on these promising feelings that live in the Ultimate Romantic Story that "makes the world go round." But you must go much deeper into the living waters of the words-and-life connection to activate them fully.*

Try looking in a mirror at the end of a long day. As you gaze at your face, repeat each of these phrases a dozen times and watch how your face changes each time: "true dignity," "quietly courageous," "sad weariness," "persevering strength," "irrepressible sparkle." See how each phrase brings a different nuance to your own face. This can show you the interactivity between the domain of suggestive ambiguity and labeling, thus the importance of eventually leaving the oversimplifications of demystified certainties. If we stay there too long, we are in danger of assuming the identity of a particular label.

Then there are the nuances of love's ever-shifting promises, as made most famous by Shakespeare's langorously romantic Duke Orsino:

> That strain again! It had a dying fall;
> O, It came o'er my ears like a sweet sound
> That breathes upon a bank of violets,
> Stealing and giving odor! Enough, no more!
> 'tis not so sweet now as it was before.
>
> TWELFTH NIGHT, I. I.

These fickle ambiguities allure by twists and unpredictable turns, forming the moment-to-moment currents in which we create, uncreate, and re-create our erotic meanings and choose our erotic actions. The details of our internal dialogue with suggestive ambiguity go on and on, down to the wire: "Can I say this, ask for this?" "Will it last afterward?" For when you put your body in the hands of another, even by the fingertips (as in tantric pariyanga), you are giving over a whole delicate web of hopes, possible embarrassments, and dreamed-upon images that, through the passions of your innocence, have made their way into your body, into your dreams, feelings, and thoughts. It is never only "sex" or "tantra" that we are having with each other. We are exposing, receiving, and touching, tentatively or boldly, each other's innocence.

If we try to ignore such alluring subtleties in whatever form they may arise, we risk cutting ourselves off from the seed-mysteries that reverberate everywhere. Then the ars erotica practices of yoga devolve into cut-and-dried how-to exercises. If we stay in the realm of flirting, the boilerplate ideas of new age clichés and scientia desire-sexuality can take hold and foreclose the entheogenic rasa maturations. And since modern sexology and psychology do not map lifelong maturation, we feel our little egos must make the whole trip. That is why we quake, causing others to quake, and then others, as well, in tense dramas that are amplified in movies and soap operas.

If we do not awaken the charismatic pathways (which are barely known in modern cultures), and instead quake only with debilitating fears, we can quickly fall into cynical certainties or cling to some demystified certainties. With the map and yogas of urdhvaretas, we can instead be invigorated to mature and become equal to a whole lifetime of challenge in which we can become holy to one another in myriad ways.

Indeed, anxiety or angst, as term-coiner Søren Kierkegaard first meant it, is the feeling that matures us, after we take "leaps of faith" into life, into "believing." Yoga adds the insight that, as our concentration "leaps" from chakra to chakra, the feeling of angst settles in each chakra for a while and matures each energy center a little further into its own blossoming. Adding mantras for each chakra adds more faith and ars erotica wisdom. Thus, our anxieties and concerns can "grow us up" into the yogic faith of chakra-maturity known as *shraddha*.

Evanescent Subtlety:
The Living Passage of Erotic Life

Going beyond the hopeless certainties of cynicism, the championing certainties of demystifying simplifications, the shimmering allure of suggestive ambiguity, we come to innocent erotic wonder, fleeting-in-this-moment, reviving-in-the-next. God-Dionysus, chief celebrant of these elusive living mysteries, of the ever-renewing springtime revelries (which, contrary to modern opinion, were not "sex orgies") warned Pentheus, representative of demystifying order and accusational authority, not to try to trap his primordial vitalism in Pentheus's stultifying grip.

> Pentheus: Seize him! This man is taunting me and Thebes.
> Dionysus: Don't bind me I tell you. You need control, not I. . . .
> He was binding me—he thought—yet he neither grasped me nor touched me. Hope was all he fed upon.
>
> EURIPIDES,
> *THE BACCHAE*

In our next movement toward mystery, the ambiguous yet compelling communications of suggestiveness dissolve in the allure of the unknown future and fascination with living impermanence. Even the exciting realm of erotic fantasies and beguiling innuendos seems like a dreaminess compared to these more vivid yet imperiled and eye-glistening beauties, mercurial blushing charms, and primordial longings.

Gaze with your partner at one another or feel each other's pulse in silence for ten or twenty minutes—it's right there, the fleeting and returning mystery.

In the opening stanzas of the *Tao Te Ching,* Lao-tzu describes this entranceway, deeper and more refined than the suggestive innuendo:

> Where the Mystery is the deepest is the gate of all that is subtle and wonderful.

Wholly temporal, erotic mystery is in the infinity of details and nuances revealed in our ever-changing, unfolding-into-the-yet-to-be contact with each other. No wonder we want to hold onto each other; no wonder we reproduce ourselves in "sexual embrace"—the mortal urgencies of time passing, not some bio-instinct, is in our very blood and marrow.

🌱 Walk quickly up a flight of stairs and then look into a mirror, or sit across from a partner and allow your heartbeat to pulse freely in your relaxed face and eyes as you gaze out. The visual world will pulse, pulse with your own living currents. In a few minutes, you will begin to see the pulsings of life in your own face in the mirror or in your partner's face. Think, "This moment goes, another comes, this moment goes. . . ." Spellbound, realize, "This is the passage of each unique moment of our ever-moving-into-the-unknown lives." Note how this comment brings out a poignant beauty in your mirrored self, or in your partner, who sees you likewise. Thus your partner's face, like a living, interactive mirror, reflects your poignancy back to you and you spontaneously respond with yet another blush, then so does your partner, and then and then. . . .

It is in our constantly deepening, temporalized, and detailed perceptions, not through some unconscious drive, that we experience the intimate and spiraling mystery of beautifying and re-creating each other. Erotic intimacy is a matter of penetrating all generalized perceptions, opinionated characterizations, excited fantasies, and, finally, our distractions to enter the unbroken flow of impermanence, until, ultimately, some incomprehensible duration after one's last breath and heartbeat, into *that Mystery*. Shared—deeply shared and ever-passing beyond our grasp—impermanence is the serpentine fundament of the erotic: that which allures us mysteriously by seeming to slip away from us while also beckoning us anew. Such soul-stirring intimacy is the result of touching beneath the stories, issues, and patterns of the relationship to each other's utterly unique, aging, re-creating, and one-day-dying presence here.

The limitations of money, time, space, family compromises, and human mortality can be enough to cascade partners into cynical certainties of fear and darkness. Or we can uplift these mundane matters into a spirituality of respect, sharing, and gratitude that is equal to the ultimate stakes of fleeting impermanence that too often threaten to overtake love: fights over money, sharing work and decisions, and all the rest.

Thus, as a therapist, I see noble struggles within trying situations—

drug addiction, affairs or "am I lovable?" insecurities—beneath any labels of "dysfunctional families." Indeed, I once guided a counselor intern in uplifting a two-generation incest-laden family from heart-rending perpetrator apologies and victim's forgiveness to planning a whole-family picnic, within a three-hour family therapy session, as the intervening courts looked on, as amazed as I was. Every few years, I check in with that counselor to be sure all this really happened, and she assures me each time that, indeed, it did.

> Try sitting across from your partner, lightly touching fingertips, and begin to gaze at each other. Think to yourselves: "This person cannot be explained. His presence is a living miracle. This is the only one of him there is, and this, now, is the one, evanescent passage of our life-mystery together. That look of tender awe in his eyes is living vulnerability and innocent courage. He sees me seeing this in him; his eyes wince. My awe is tinged with fear of unknown possibilities of each and all the next moments. My fear is soothed by the sharing. I feel tingling in us, an echoing into the future of new lives. We are singular mortals and, yet, possibly more."
>
> Even as you separate and close your eyes, be careful not to misinterpret the experience of slipping-by impermanence as "abandonment," especially at times of saying goodbye to someone you love. Impermanence is heightened at such times, but no one is causing it, discarding us, or abandoning us. All moments pass and, blamelessly, we are always saying goodbye to the impermanent present and hello to the unknown future. Such are the constant poignancies of erotic evanescence.

To see someone following the shifting glimmers of our never-happened-before self will always present us with a daring and blame-lessly difficult paradox. We are both totally allured and hard-pressed not to turn away in shy trepidation or sudden awe of what we see and of being seen so profoundly. Like any mystery, erotic intimacy seems elusive, softly beckoning us with no little quaking, for evanescent subtlety is the entrance to "where the mystery is the deepest." Beth describes the heightened closeness that she and Gary discover in the subtleties of feeling that, ironically, live most poignantly in the moments when they turn away from each other:

> *We were talking about moving in with each other, marriage and family. At first, I was angry and disappointed in Gary because he seemed afraid to really commit to the relationship. Then I saw that it is because he had invested so much meaning in our possibly having a future together that he was sort of overwhelmed by the possibilities, as was I. When he told me of his roller coaster of feelings, I realized how very involved with me he was. I started to feel that we really are in the same uncertainty of life, together.*
>
> *I realized that I had been shyly turning away from him at the very moment his feelings of hopeful uncertainty would be the strongest because, in seeing him that way, my own similar feelings would seem unbearable. And the same was true for Gary. He would see my hopes and fears rise and would bashfully turn away in the moment just as they peaked.*
>
> *Then we began sharing these "turning point feelings" without turning away at the last moment, not as listeners and speakers but in a silent meditation. We began experiencing this amazing flow of feelings that, ironically, was always being disrupted by our talking about our feelings, or in that most critical moment when we would actually turn away from each other. I felt a spiritual quality, a faith in each other, that the divine is real and eternal. We were in some kind of time flow.*
>
> *Through the meditation, we shared the ride we were already on, rather than fighting about who was to blame for the hilly parts of the ride. Sharing our fears this way converted our blamings and differences into precarious yet intimate unions.*

In this vignette, what is often pathologized as a fear of intimacy emerges under closer examination as a plethora of fluctuations and innuendos that, fortunately, no amount of "clear communication" or assertiveness can dispel. Only by devotedly paying attention to each fleeting moment do we deepen this kind of intimacy. We see and share this existential-erotic mystery in our quivering, not in spite of it or by subduing it, and certainly not in our personalized guilts and blamings. That we are mortal is no one's fault. The depths to which we mature more and more, year after year, decade after decade, must be given ensouled ars erotica bodies, far beyond the maps of the scientia sexualis.

The endearing blush of self-consciousness as we just look at each other begins to reveal this fragile yet utterly charming rapport. Somewhat uncomfortably embarrassed, we want to look away and have often used a seductive move, or even an argument, to do so. But if we refrain, we can begin to share these feelings of the impermanent, more vulnerable self, stirring myriad unnameable passions before our most heartfelt meditative regard.

In this phenomenology of impermanence, that most innocent of feelings, shyness (and its pink nuances of embarrassment; azures of an alluring coyness; silvers of over-delight; rosy, hoped-for acceptance; brazen, yet trepid curiosity; and, once purged of popular pejorations, many dark-velvety folds of shame) is the wavering eminence of the now concealing, now revealing soul and serves as the emotional illuminant for all greater being-in-the-world.

By this point, the spellbound gatekeeper of focused awareness has given up all of her cynicisms, demystified certainties, and exciting imaginings. To continue, she gives up even her rapt wonderings that sparkle and fade, again and again. She now aspires toward the inspired awe of romantic-poetic revelations, meditation, and surrendered spontaneous worship.

In the ars erotica, couples feel challenged to become comfortable hearing or saying such things as: "I revere you. You are beyond the beyond. I can taste the taste of you from here and you taste like fire and jasmine. I feel so happy, I might cry. The smell of your yoni, your breasts, the allure of your neck where your pulse surges and vanishes is making me high, stop it, no, more, *more*. It's all so perfect. Your eyes are blossoming like prowling tigers, your arms are like a summer breeze all over me, your heart is as glowing and welcoming as the Home of all homes, the Wish of all wishes, the Birth of every birth."

Such sentimental, even poetic expressions often require getting over shyness or feeling too corny or unfamiliar. We might feel we are giving up a whole life-mode of cynicism, sarcastic humor, and bashfulness and going into mushland. But when you are together in this fleeting romantic realm that reemerges from time passage itself, you just might say all such things, in spite of yourselves. If not, at the very end, most of us will surely wish we had, and more. Thus, the Grand Yogaverse says we reincarnate back to new births to "do better next time and the next and the next."

Meditative Knowing:
Entering the Intimus

In the steadied gaze resulting from spellbound rapture in the heart of our existence, some might say, "We are in the hands of deity. This is a miracle. I see you as sixteen and glowing, as twenty and vibrant, as one hundred and radiant with the soul's beauty." Others will merely grow silent and trace the pulses in your veins as they surge and vanish. Rasa, entheogenic experiences, emerge that need no further confirmation, that grow profusely and wildly (that is, innocently) from within ars erotica bodies and the souls that "ensoul" them.

Like the softly arriving first light of morning stars that soothes this wrinkled earth unfailingly just before each dawn, the etheric glow of the soul emerges as the undying and merciful sentience within each other's eyes, and yet is beyond that. For this primordial witness to all realities is both within and beyond sight, hearing, touch, and life and death.

Infinities of impossibly weathered times and immeasurable joys have left their mark as the muted receptivity just behind the eyes' sparkle. But behind, before, and after all the events of life that have affected us—in the eyes and souls of the newborn, to be sure, but also in those of the aged and dying, the quiet neighbor, the impassioned artist, and even the sullen criminal—are dark pools of eternity; this is the inscrutable liquid depth from which all lives emerge and into which all converge. In this inner sanctum, a meditative intimacy yields to reverence and worshipfulness and urdhvaretas fructifies as unencumbered and unswervingly as the sperm-ovum union of two twenty-five-year-olds conceiving madly, as divinely guided as Mother's gestational, incarnating movements.

High and bemused one afternoon,
we dreamed a dream of going off
blending into the trees wind streams
churning the hours the months lost
in the upward igniting of bodies within bodies
each body waiting for us to devote everything,
for that's what it takes,
what eight hours a day are for.
One day the pineal cocoon engorges cock erect,
takes off her shirt nipples forth,
sunbursts inwardly blinding
like that first emission or menses everything suddenly
changed from one moment to the next
gone forth beyond mere fertility
flooding the full-moon suffusing everywhere
radiating into the permeating world
imbuing the living dharma*
while all else grows hazy and remote,
we in the thick of it
the fecund mystery of incarnation
undistracted
making each other real.

Far beyond the "deployment of sex," these hidden ars erotica passions begin to flower in earnest within the surrendered, meditative intimus as mudras and asanas, as shaktipat activations, trance dancing as ecstatically alive while "gone from this world," rasas dripping down the corners of your mouth. Your eyes become orbs of gratitude, your bones breathe invisibly down to the very marrow, which sings with newly born blood cells, all bathing you in their nourishing, red pulsing warmth. Testes and ovary follicles quiver like a million scintillating star flecks singing a midnight gamelan of infinite splendors.

Dharma is a way, or manner, of life or of acting in a particular situation that is in accord with spiritual principles.

Within the lifelong inner marriage of the advanced kundalini-awakened yogi, the ars erotica puberties described in sacred yogic texts manifest wildly; that is, as naturally as bee-intoxicating wildflowers in summer's heat:

When, with spellbound awe over thousands of hours of yoga practice one's whole being has matured, there arises effortlessly of its own accord a natural tumescence that moves one heel into the perineum and the other heel above the genitals in the equipoise of "conjoined-matured cosmic powers" (*siddha-asana*) and then the tumescence of the triple lock—the root lock of the closed anal-perineal muscles [violet-edged perineum, *mula bandha*), the flying-up lock [under the lungs diaphragmatic tumescence, *uddiyana bandha*], and the water-holder lock [chin-pressed-to-chest, brachial-swelling-veins-tumescence, *jalandhara bandha*]—also occurs in this natural way. There is no other tumescence like the *siddha-asana* tumescence, no other mindspace than the embryonic mindspace become fully wizened and mature, no other delight gesture like the tongue-to-pineal tumescence [*khechari mudra*], and no other charismatic beauty like the blossoming of ubiquitous divine ecstatic sound-feelings [*anahata-nad*].[1]

3

Shared-Gender Mystery

Of the many provocative sexological redefinitions that emerge from an understanding of eros as mystery, perhaps none is more fascinating than the notion that gender does not exist except as a shared elastic interdependency. In this light gender is seen as the fundamental condition of erotic embodiment that men and women find themselves in, rather than as a way to differentiate one from the other, or even to distinguish the specific behavioral patterns each displays toward the other. We will be entering gender as a mystery being shared.

Gender names that class of human phenomena that includes friend, partner, rival, and enemy. Like friendship or rivalry, gender reverberates *between* people, not in them. Gender always implies (with infinitely more cogency than the less alluring term *selfhood*) a mystery of ever more subtle rapports going on with another and with the world.

Gender is also a subject heading, as in "gender issues." Only one other heading grasps as fully the integration of all constituent elements under its rubric, and that is the heading "ecology." For example, while *forest* is a one-dimensional name for "an expanse of wilderness," the term *forest ecology* is a multidimensional name that denotes an exceedingly dynamic interactivity and ever-refinable relatedness, even synchronous oneness. Change one branch, and changes ripple throughout the entire forest ecology.

Likewise, people may share many things (history, language, religion, culture), but when we refer to them as *gendered people,* their dimensionality suddenly and exponentially ramifies. Suddenly the sense of an elusive, shared mystery drifts among them (as it does in the ecology of a forest community). To understand gender, watch the more suggestive, subtle, and mysterious sharings among people (or any other life forms).

Gender is like the water two fish swim in that makes their play with each other visible and possible. It is the play or shared interaction of any two or more people regarding erotic mystery. Even our physiologies change distinctly and sometimes dramatically when we live with, or separate from, a lover. A definition of gender that distinguishes the composite traits of male-bodied persons from the composite traits of female-bodied persons (that is, *gender* as specifying gender *differences*) is very persuasive but is insufficient to deal with the interactive reality of gender.

MALE AND FEMALE AS STARTING POINTS

The terms *female* and *male* are merely starting points in the life of gender and imply a relatedness between a man and a woman or between two women or two men that is different than the relatedness between a twenty-year-old person and a thirty-year-old person. Reading a story about a person, rather than about a man or a woman, provokes scant erotic mystery in the reader (except in the way that the term *person* is itself an alluring veil).

But as soon as we say that a woman reads a story about some person, a little more of the erotic mystery begins to stir. And then the person in the story turns out to be a man. But then the woman reader is a lesbian, while the story-male, as in a Shakespearean drama, is really a woman. A woman who is attracted to . . . we can go on and on tracking the crests and falls of shared-gender permutations in which *male* and *female* are purely suggestive of something or other but are meaningless in themselves—in an inevitable and inescapable process of shifting nuances, possibilities, and plot swervings.

I can think of no more tragic an example of the scientia sexualis mission of assigning each person a proper gender (even the liberal attempts at LGBTTQI categorizations retain this trope) than as can be seen in the diary of the nineteenth-century hermaphrodite, Herculine Barbin, written at the time when the medical scientia profession first took up this categorizing task. Brought into contemporary awareness via its publication and commentary by Michel Foucault, the reader of Herculine's diary traces the innocent frivolity of female-seeming Herculine among her young girl students suddenly anatomically "examined" and "determined to be a man," whereafter Herculine's story is amplified and spun through the sensationalizing tabloid journalism of its times, she is fired, suffers a complete mental breakdown, and commits suicide.

GENDER IS THE SHARING OF MYSTERY

Gender is itself the sharing of mystery. Gender is something we are immersed in profoundly, and mystery is the experience of profound immersion in an alluring uncanniness. This is the particular beauty of the term *gender:* It points to the erotic immersion that we all share. Just walk down a busy street and feel the interactivity of gender mystery. Feel the awe, suspense, curiosity, and spontaneous allure—cues that we are immersed in a shared mystery.

As we shall see, our erroneous conventional understanding of "separate genders" or gender as gender *differences* is the fault line of anguished tumult between men and women in our contemporary erotic world. Our problems with gender are fundamentally conceptual and then perceptual; we have expunged sharedness from the concept of gender and have expunged mystery from our too certain perceptions of sharing and being. Only a contacting of one another in careful wonder can re-reveal "sharing" and "gender" as indivisible.

To understand sharing is to understand gender, but it is not the active-voice transitive verb, as in "He shared his seat with her" or "She shared her ideas with him" or even "They shared their resources with each other." The sharing I have in mind is not wielded by anyone, for the sharing of gender is a fully interactive *condition* that we, as men and women, find ourselves in, not a set of stable traits or behaviors inherent to one or the other.

Sharing is the realization or perception that with reference to gender, men and women are in an ecological or "same boat" situation with one another. It is this realization that provokes a sense of awe, dread, relief, or respect, for shared interactive gender makes us inherently committed to one another. The inescapability and the equal degree of being in this gendered condition are what make it a shared condition. Gender, like procreativity, is an inexplicable trust given to us. It is a trust in the sense of being a reservoir of possibility, as in a trust fund. As well, it is trust as a magnetlike, inherent holding together, felt as an uncanny connectedness, an allure, a hope, and, most certainly, a need.

If the criterion for being a romantic-erotically lovable and loving person were to be ars erotica entheogenic maturity, then such would become the basis of cultural erotic sharing, en masse, for that culture and scientia sexualis would fade into the "old way" that people "used to share gender."

Sharing Lost . . .

Even if men and women speak and act as if gender is not an utterly shared trust, we are still in it as our given condition. We then share the lack of this recognition. We share it just as blacks and whites, Arabs and Jews, rich and poor must share any lack of recognizing certain truths regarding the shared human trust called specieshood. The problems that emerge in such contradictions breed in the contorted but unavoidable sharedness that still remains.

If one boat mate says to the other that she is not getting what she needs from the other, what she is doing with the shared condition is seeing a problem and announcing it. The two now share (intransitively) and interact regarding the complaint "My needs aren't being met."

The deeper problem for this pair is that the sense of sharing the same boat on the same deep waters is in jeopardy of being swamped by the emotions stirred by the complaint. What if they lose sight of the irrevocable sharedness of their situation and think the *single* thing they share and now must do something about is the declared problem of an unmet need? What happens? The way of differences unfolds.

Gradually they will come to believe that they are not in the same boat at all, not even clinging to its turned-over sides together. They begin to think and feel and speak to each other as if they are in different universes. Instead of sharing this dubious feeling of being in different universes, they start to measure and dogmatize their observed differences, perhaps as gender-based, irresolvable differences, and wonder if they have ever shared anything but differences! They then start to live as if they are in two separate universes, reaching over the wall to make any contact. Thus devolves the vivisection of the shared-gender mystery. In the gaping expanse of this preoccupation with differences, dark fears seem to look back at us. What Jung termed our own "shadow" meets us.

Disparities in societal opportunities solidify; moods of superiority-inferiority infect. The beauties and risks of flirtation become suspect, exploited, and compromised. The significance of gender itself feels so insufficient that men and women resort to exaggerated mythic images—the "wild-men," the "wolf-women." Love itself feels so dangerous that authorities apply the concepts of addiction to much of romantic life—and they are believed, as the proliferation of (gender-based) support groups testifies. As the fluid play of shared gender rigidifies, we lose some of our sense of humor and political correctness, moralism and ensuing fears of "men" and of "women" lock in as each jolts, seeing the other's look of suspicion aimed at himself or herself and peering back out of one's own eyes. Even the eye-quavering looks of desire and allure *seem* dangerous. Indeed, the innate safety that otherwise comes from mutual gender respect before each other as life-creating mysteries seems to be thousands of impossible miles away. I suddenly recall, decades ago, being in a remote village in India. A ten-year-old girl appears out of nowhere, innocently starts dancing classical Indian movements and singing in front of me and an Indian man as we chat on a park bench; she smiles at us and dances away. Thousands of miles away from these modern, fraught, and fearful scientia sexualis times, indeed!

Homophobia emerges where compassion fails regarding HIV. Not a single new thought on the abortion debate emerges; instead, battle lines are drawn more deeply. A symptomatology of divorce, rape, batterings, misanthropy and misogyny, and victimhood precipitates. Millions of people recount painful memories of childhood sexual abuse, numberless others report incidents of sexual harassment, and in this confusion still others retract specious complaints based on false memories of sexual abuse.

. . . Sharing Found

Certainly the final mapping of the phenomena of gender (and the solutions to the above conundrums) will not come through yet another investigation of the differences between men and women. The map, and solutions of any depth, will come only through the comprehensive study of gender as a conjoint and mysterious sharing of erotic powers, for that is what gender is. Framing the research question in terms of contrast, such as, "What are the differences between men's and women's abilities, linguistics, or attributes?" ruptures the in vivo phenomenon that is being approached.

Adherents of these findings on why women are thus and men are different at first feel empowered by their "verified" specificity. They enjoy the explanatory power of the discovered differences and employ this information in daily life with hopeful conviction. Later, which for our culture is now, they begin to feel the limitations of these gender objectifications: the stereotypes are discerned and resisted; the panacea fails to deliver. In spite of all the best-selling reports and studies, the demystifying method guaranteed as much from the onset, for these findings are often little more than shadow measurements in the proverbial Platonic cave.

Those who would study gender as a shared reality, like those who would attempt to feel the heat of the Burning Bush, struggle with more mysterious problems outside the cave, in the dizzying radiance of living gender powers. In the ars erotica, every solution to a problem of gender spirals into a more intricate sense of sharing.

The question must be asked, "Why might individuals want to define genders based on differences?" The answer will inevitably imply difficulties with sharing, overdetermining theories of "individuation," entrenched cynical certainties, and a fear or denial of even fleeting spiritual responses to the other. Such difficulties are not a function of gender differences but of the uncanniness of sharing uncertainty, suggestivity, subtlety, and mystery. Questionings intoned one way will seem to lead us to convincing literal answers, or intoned another way, to awesome experiences of the incomprehensible. The former emerge from scientia sexualis, the latter from ars erotica. We must recover through intimate and artful means the wonder *of,* not information *about,* one another. Awe, not certainty, signals that we are gaining knowledge about gender.

Even our "own" gender is inextricably rooted in the combination of our two parents' gametes, while the seeds of our children's possible lives tingle mysteriously in our bodies, awaiting deeper contact with the seed of some other. The biological believe-it-or-nots of gender amorphousness— the hermaphroditic phase of normal embryological development, the rare but real adult hermaphrodites, and the various gender transmutations of the greater plant and animal world—should give us some pause. Heterosexuals fail to learn anything new about the fluidity of gender from gay, lesbian, bisexual, and transgendered persons. One wonders if we will ever leave the shallows of "sort-and-file" gender enframement for the more mysterious depths of an utterly shared gender.

Even our observations of other cultures and species have been made through these gross lenses. Monkeys grooming and preening one another, the vast array of animal mating behaviors and rituals, and the cross-cultural diversity of social-erotic customs are best described as an ever-changing, interactive play of gender, not as "male behavior" and "female behavior," nor as a primordial scientia sexualis polyamory. But the scientist of gender asserts, "The female always does the x behavior, and the male always does the $1/x$ behavior; therefore, there are two distinct genders." No: x and $1/x$ are functions of each other; they are mutually variable with regard to each other and thus determine each other at unfathomable levels of pheromonal and interactive rasa subtlety.

Even the idea that each person can be pegged on some kind of continuum from ultramasculinity to ultrafemininity is only relatively useful. Androgyny, the synthesis of masculine and feminine qualities in any person, still locates gender within a sort of psychic bisexuality and is only a symbol for the living condition of shared gender. The principles of social systems theory, in which roles and meanings are understood as group phenomena, can provide some insight into the fact that the significance of a person's gender is shared by the group, but not strongly enough to make the radical leap we now approach.

What we are looking for is a fundamental ecology of gender and a romantic and erotic sense of this ecology in our relationships. For shared gender is not just a partnership, as Riane Eisler proposes in *The Chalice and the Blade*. This cooperative, same-team metaphor misses the profundity of how deeply and indistinguishably the roots of gender entwine and tendril into the ground of our existence.

Partners who cooperate together, who get paid equally, and who worship goddesses as well as gods might never know in their bones how very *shared* and alchemically, reverberatingly, and mutually empowering the condition of human gender is despite the intermingling closeness that sexual intercourse inherently *is*. The kind of knowledge of each other that I am speaking of is different from all of that. It is a knowing that is verified when it *provokes* a spiritual response of each to the other: a mood of devotion and reverence that trails into shy astonishment and ever-more-empowering displays of passion, with the entheogenic response of allowing our lover to make us feel we are completely beside ourselves, witnessing god or goddess in human form sitting there radiating all the charms of the universe before our very eyes, loving us with a love supreme, evoking play-of-the-gods dances in romantic-erotic repartee, ars erotica actions, grihastha home creations within the shared confidence of "Yes, yes, yes, till death do us part and again, yes!"

> *Really mean it till death do us part:*
> *Holding your wrists you writhe slightly this way then that*
> *your outer surfaces contiguous with the invisible realms*
>   *of you*
> *giving rise to a path leading to surrenders*
> *you squeezed my hand I give up, your hips raise to one side*
> *you bite gently your own lower lip press your finger*
> *as if to silence the gasp of it all fainting into yourself*
> *into the infinity of the future uplifted into a haze*
> *we entered the subtle realm where starry everything glows.*

Each preferring to give, nothing was ever lost,
stretching ourselves thin for one another we became vast.
Easing the way for me for you as the decades wandered on
no sorrow or illness endured alone,
parents aging before us and dying, friends passing, all
*   eventually pass.*
When you squeezed my hand hard and held it there
the day I got that dreaded call, I will never forget it—
I am here, you said, I am not going anywhere,
and when my grip weakens, then my gaze upon you will
*   lock,*
when that at last should blur,
then resolute in my heart shall you remain,
your name the last sound on my lips,
your lips the last image in my mind . . .

While give-and-take partnering and cooperation is a common understanding of sharing, it falls short of perceiving gender as a shared *mysterious* reality and then living up to that perception. All such concepts as give and take belong to the materialistic realm of economic exchange and fail to settle into the more ontological potencies from which gender manifests—the spiritual economy: *nemein,* a disbursing sharing, within the intimate place of sharing, *oikos,* the home.

Instead of wonder and awe at the reality of shared gender, we usually seek literal answers to our questions about this mystery. We believe knowledge comes from demystification, which, in the domains of eros, can be fatal. In our current world—where eros is demystified as ultimately meaning a well-defined desire—gender definitions turn out to be what we want genders to be like. Gender gets caught in desirability, and its mystery is shaped likewise.

We do not relate to gender as shared mystery but as specific need-fulfilling commodities (we are to "meet needs"), explanatory resources, and vested-interest groups. We think of gender as a given that can be used to explain why things are the way they are; it's this way because of men, because of women; the one must change; the other; no, both must change.

The historical record reveals our difficulties with gender and the sharing of social power, but not the more subtle spiritual history of the fall of gender-as-shared-mystery into gender-as-assignable-differences. In "tantric genderosophy," we see that we do in fact call forth or limit the possibilities for one another's gender (for any particular time span). Yet tantra takes its stand upon gender as a shared mystery, the recovery of which provokes an inherent awe and spiritual respectfulness of one another. Such provocative spiritual knowledge can form the basis for social and political revisions, just as the plea for a "deep"—that is, spiritually provocative—ecological vision can provide the internal motivation for needed environmental protections.

GENDER AWE

The inequities between the genders, currently discussed as the history of patriarchal dominance and sexism, cannot be reversed merely through scholarly research, as some might hope, nor through political initiatives, as many demand. Spiritual problems, even if they also foster material inequities, require spiritual solutions. Sanctity can be neither proved nor legislated and lies beyond anyone's political agenda. Reverence is always an unrequested response to another who is perceived as being beyond all of our scientia concepts and estimations. We must let the other mean that much to us. Typically, forgiveness, contrition, and reconciliation wash through worshippers in these moments as well. Such is the transformative potency of a spiritual resource.

Certainly, reverence does not belong more to the one gender than to the other, nor does it belong to those who worship gods rather than goddesses. For it is not the form or gender of the deity that matters but the depth of the reverence its devotees bestow upon it.

If reverence be profound and ever-spreading of its blessings, one can worship a cobblestone—humility may, after all, be divine. We can recover the birthright or trust given us as gendered creatures only through the holy recognition of an utterly shared gender.

These feelings are not some kind of rare luxury that only a few select individuals deserve, nor are they rarefied emotions to be reserved for special occasions. The situation is in fact the reverse: reverence is the *only* sentiment we do not earn. It is the universal response to the other as the mystery that she or he is, just for being "the other," the starting point for ars erotica mutually provocative wonders.

This is the deepest erotic opportunity we provide each other: to be humbled and exalted reciprocally. Quietly watch the other's sleeping face for one minute. The mystery is not far away. This overlooked nearness is our tragedy.

As for reverence being a luxury, would that were true, for whatever we shy away from worshipping inevitably atrophies and lives on in an ever more withering state. Thus the future of gender is itself at stake, and it shows. We have turned away from the deep beauty of one another and no longer worship one another or the earth we walk on. Instead, we rest upon the "surface" tumescences of desirability, shying away from those arousals of awe and surrender. Only worship of one another is profound enough to call forth the deepest of human possibilities, and only the depths of possibility provoke our awe. In erotic reality, possibility and mystery stand higher—have more alluring "life" in them—than actuality and certainty.

Admiring one another, struggling and accomplishing together, come and go as talents, crises, and projects come and go. These are responses to life's actualities. They are well worth exploring with one another. But more alluringly mysterious is the reverence for another essentially because she or he is *other,* because dawning in the other are living, yet uncertain possibilities. Self-worship is viable, but only in the same way another can worship us: we must stand back in awe, humbled by the inherent holiness we radiate upon one another. We can create or at least nurture life and have been created by seed forces that genetic science can trace but not explain. We come from something very, very Deep.

GENDER WORSHIP

Worship is what even the immortals long to do, and they willingly relinquish their immortality in order to find something to bow to. What they long to worship is the other, not themselves. Thus, the immortals become the other—that is, mortals—in order to carry out their sacred rites. They become us, we become them, over and over again.

यत्र नार्यस्तु पूज्यन्ते तत्र रमन्ते देवताः

"Where man/woman is worshipped is the play of the Divine"

This is the crowning touch to a recentering of eros with mystery: We discover through a devotional meditation, or other such means, that, erotically, we are in a shared mystery together, that all the psychological interpretations, desires, fears, and expectations we have about each other merely circulate around the inexplicable mystery that every man or woman is.

> *"Filled with joy"* is such a ringing singing phrase.
> *Like shiny brass turquoise and garnet bejeweled Tibetan*
>   *icon couples*
> *in upright thrilled embrace, blossoming in those icons*
> *secret truths mystico-erotica original religion*
> *fully-matured upward inward all glands alive tumescent*
>   *engorged*
> *totally intent the one upon the other*
> *perfectly in love*
> *designed by the cosmos*
> *each quantum crystal species plant animal male and*
>   *female*
> *to capture the full attention*
> *the one of the other the other of the one*
> *in perfect symmetry.*

If we are unsure whether our devotion is authentic, we must take it on faith that it is, for it is greater than we are at those times. Our worship of each other will frequently be a mystery to us, particularly when we don't believe this is possible. In such uncertainty the mystery has a chance to grow, our faith has a chance to grow.

We also allow ourselves to be worshipped, not as a great person but as mystery; that is, for reasons we may know nothing about and must therefore take on faith. Meditative worship is the opportunity for each of us to transcend our conditioned beliefs about each other for some moments, even amid the most trying times of a marriage or relationship, and to experience the mystery that lives in spite of the dramas and crises. It is a return to the possible as real and to the hidden as a promise. Thus we recover the reverence that can be obscured by fearfulness.

Worship is merely the response to the perceived erotic truth of the other and not a strategy to some further ends. It is certainly not a requirement, like routine church attendance. It is the most profound and enigmatic expression of the shared-gender mystery. And charismatically shaking, playfully wild, seed-rasa-mudra-activating worship contains its own overwhelming motivation to attend the Church of Endless Ars Erotica.

Whether the privilege of worship rests with the worshipped or the worshipper is altogether unclear; it is even unclear whether there are such distinctions at the core of the shared-gender mystery. As you will see, the love-making practices of tantric brahmacharya hover in this uncertainty, in the partners' ever more vulnerable and empowering intimacy with each other. As you discover worship of each other in some mundane moment, such as when doing the dishes, watching TV, or feeling resentful, you will go even deeper into this tantric paradox of holiness hidden everywhere.

The seeming risk is for the partner who makes the *first* offering to the other, without any concern for reciprocation but merely as the *immediate recognition* of the holy mystery of the other and the opportunity this holiness provides for us, originally and eternally. When we contact the erotically worshipful in each other, we must face the ironic fact that it has always been there and in ourselves as well.

THE PROSTHESIS OF AN OWNED SEXUALITY

Even the notion of one's "own" sexuality is a politicized derivation or appropriation of eros, a personal act through which one hopes to attain a sense of being an autonomous agent. As a collective, public act, the proclamation of an ownable and owned sexuality is intended to redress previous inequities by producing socially recognized personhood, as in the inspirational slogans "Woman Power" and "Gay Power."

We would like to own various powers, and popular psychology supports these aspirations with its encouragements to "reclaim" or "own your sexuality." But the erotic powers of sexuality—love, attraction, arousal, fertility, families, and surrender—are entrusted to us or, rather, among us and are not "owned." Such slogans are merely transitional metaphors or therapeutic word tools to help us recover from domestic violence, depression, social-political abuse, low self-esteem, or drug addiction (in which heroin and amphetamines play the role of the greatest rip-off artist of ars erotica's natural ecstatic chemistries for users and of the ever-forgiving loyalty chemistries of their "codependent" closest ones) or alcoholism (in which alcohol is rasa rip-off artist number two).

Such terms belong to the technologies of recovery and rehabilitation. Although the image of an owned sexuality can be a temporarily effective prosthetic word tool, it should not be used in mapping the intimate contours of erotic space, for prostheses and maps serve entirely different functions. After we have recovered, we must put away such prosthetic devices, for we cannot pass through the eye of the needle of intimacy carrying our own sexuality with us. When two give to one another, love becomes infinite.

We are for ourselves best when we are for each other,
a lifelong exploration of the preposition for
humble overlooked what are things for
a yearning, I am in love with for,
giver beyond myself bowing, finally, in devotion
each other granting exquisiteness to each other,
really meaning it,

becoming symbiotic with you, source of my awe.
Orienting the minutes hours toward you,
the purpose to get up early to listen to you breathe,
as the day finally ends racing stop lights to get to you,
you say when I don't know what else to say I say, you you
I say yes yes.

It might be just as helpful for some people to hear that they needn't worry about owning a sexuality or not owning one. Often in such cases when people have suffered abuse, they need merely to learn how and when to say "no" or "yes" to others within the context of the shared-gender mystery. The deeper goal implied by this quest for "personal power" or "reclaimed sexuality" seems to be respect, and an appeal to surrender to an ecological embeddedness of all relationships (especially those of romantic love and family life of children, grandchildren, and grandparents and so on) in the Whole.

Respect for each other is most authentic when it is a secondary response to feeling the awe and vulnerability of the other or oneself. Respect for our own erotic nature is a matter of being moved by the lyrical romanticism—the spirit—of life that we, as humans, are entrusted with, as our collectively shared and interactive nature. When charismatically energized, respect for one another gives back one hundredfold in mutual entheogenic rasa interactivities. We become god/goddess dancing endlessly with one another.

No one owns any part of nature's spirit or its powers and beauties. If we can discover the poetry of nature (human-erotic and otherwise), what it is we seek through "owning" it or "reclaiming" it will have been accomplished: a kind of ecological—that is, respectfully shared—balance of self-and-others, of humanity-in-the-world, that will always remain somewhat beyond our control, as mystery. In fully matured conjugal urdhvaretas, the power of the shared-gender mystery unlocks ars erotic heat that owned sexualities cannot ignite.

In the rough-and-tumble world, arming ourselves with the idea of an owned sexuality and gender may feel like an attractive strategy. The more you feel you "own" your "own sexuality," the easier it is to divorce or break up and pack up and leave; thus, prenuptial agreements seem like a self-protective "good idea." The less that children are understood as being born of the flesh of "two become as one flesh," the easier it is to see "split-time, coparenting" as a reasonable and ever more common parental structure. Yes, as an over correction for the church's scientia of sacrificial love, self-affirming and more calculating scientia sexualis psychologies have been fashioned, with good cause, since we might give a lot to someone yet receive back a pittance. But as Rilke has said, "In the end it is our unshieldedness on which we depend." Unshieldedness is a sufficient stance only when we have grasped our final essence as being infinitely resourceful—that is, in our discovery that humans are souled beings. We have an ultimate meaning and innocence that cannot be taken away, for it is inseparable from us, even by death. Merciful and ever forgiven, we ring with soul. Can or will we see each other—and be seen and *feel* seen by each other, and gratefully so—as endlessly resourceful souls? And in such wholly commingled seeing-and-feeling-seen, how can we *not* but want to leap into unreserved commitments and a deeply ecological interconnectedness with one another in our romantic and familial relationships, until death do us part?

Under even the most tortuous of conditions, the soul replenishes us, not omnipotently but inexhaustively. Thus, the higher spirit of tragedy: the strange capacity to endure and live through untoward and even cruel hardships is part of the human condition. Often it is tragedy that surfaces the soul-sense as being deeper than the personality-self, the soul's everyday agent. We discover that we are more than our personalities ever thought. Popular psychology's concept of the "survivor" of past abuse is further cleansed of victimistic overtones within the spiritual psychology of soul. The soul as our essence radiates an inherent dignity untouchable by worldly abuse.

A dread accompanies grasping the awe of the soul's capacity to endure all, for the implication is that if the dreadful were to happen, we are capable of enduring it and thus we would go through such unthinkable fires, unavoidably. Such strength is not good news for the limited personality-self of psychology, and rightly so. For the limited personality-self "knows" with great terror that it cannot endure the most dreadful of possibilities.

We must know the soul to grasp the depth of such fortitude, a knowledge that would radically transform most of contemporary psychology.

Cut off from a sense of the enduring spiritual resources of the soul, our demystifying psychology has come to believe that the personality-self is best restored by creating strong boundaries around its periphery and "owning oneself." But *boundaries* is merely another prosthetic word-tool, a crutchlike means to some end; certainly it does not accurately map erotic reality.

As Martin Buber has stated, "Every *It* is bounded by others; *It* exists only through being bounded by others. But when *Thou* is spoken, there is no thing. *Thou* has no bounds."[1]

The goal is not to build boundaries but to feel respect and share it with others. This goal is better obtained by fathoming the spiritual fortitude and uncanny resilience of the awesome soul that is our essential nature. When the charismatic energies of Shiva-Shakti emerge, sharing replaces the prosthesis of "boundaries" with the profuse abundance of entheogenic co-creativity, equal to a lifetime of unbreakable sharing.

The recently coined metaphor of "soul murder" is a particularly costly overdramatization used to emphasize the horrifics of interpersonal mistreatment (and perhaps to deter future perpetrators). Unlike the body, however, the soul cannot be murdered, nor can it be "wounded" to later "survive" such blows. Devastations, abuses, and crises are obstacles that, when dealt with from the integrity of the soul, will mature and soften us—sometimes even unite us in a transformed relationship with our adversaries.

Thus, the key etymological secret power in the word *soteriology* (spiritual salvation) is *te,* which refers to tumescence, swellings that arouse the soul's power to heal oneself and become even stronger than before. The ancient Greeks knew—as did the early Christians, who also made use of this term for "redemptive healing"—that forgiveness, love and caring, apology, gratitude, faithful longing and persevering, moods of awe and humbled reverence, righteousness of any clearly justifiable outrage (such as being righteously outraged by apartheid or any unjust actions), and giving and sharing are far more important than the scientia sexualis–favored clinical emotions, the "letting out" of sheer anger (emptied of its driving reason), grief as cathartic crying (rather than lost-forever love), boundary assertion (instead of respect creation, charismatic interactivation), sex desire (instead of seed-infused, profound-pleasure creation), and so on.

While the popular clinical concept of wounding provokes a kind of pathos that leaves us less than we were, that of an encountered "obstacle" engenders a daring and suspenseful response in which we remain whole and challenged to continue to participate in our lives. Thus, we have, on one hand, the labeling of our difficulties as a wounding or a murdering, requiring a shoring up of boundaries (against the "other") and an owning of one's power (taking it back from the "other"). On the other hand we see our difficulties as obstacles that draw out the more hidden powers of our souls in unshielded living within the strangely vulnerable mystery of reciprocal awe for one another. The differences between these two linguistic routes through adversity could be all the difference in the world, for each leads to the creation of a different kind of world of selves and others. As the great linguist Ludwig Wittgenstein noted, "to imagine a language means to imagine a form of life."[2]

HOMOSEXUAL MYSTERY

From the perspective of ars erotica, we are *homosexual* as soon as we like another man or another woman. It is only through the reduction of erotic mystery to sex desire and, perhaps, to fertility that homosexuality becomes difficult for many heterosexuals to fathom. Why are men attracted to other men with a sex desire, why women to other women? For that matter, why are men and women attracted to one another?

The answer is again a matter of wonder and amazement, and psychological, biological, or religious concepts merely obfuscate the uncanniness of erotic attraction with their interpretations, research findings, and judgments. The path that seems to lead one to the persons he or she loves is as many-layered and enigmatic as the currents of the oceans.

The capacity to see beauty in another to the degree that passion arises is a sign of individual sensitivity, for it is our surrendering that makes the other attractive, as much as it is another's beauty that induces us to surrender willingly. Two men or two women can even feel the home-building passions of fertility stirred by each other within the context of their sharing of gender, as well as the passions of desire and sublimation. They may partially or openly grieve that, just as with an infertile heterosexual couple, the mystery denies them conception. They share this limitation.

Coded cues of seduction and drag disguises that reveal the "true self"; ultraguarded privacies where one's home has been a closet; one's loving as a private struggle to accept and then, one hopes, to enjoy; a "difference" from others described by them but hidden from oneself: such are a few of the ambiguities of hiddenness in the homosexual mystery.

Within the ars erotica yoga of emotions known as *bhakti* devotional yoga, gender gets even more profound and diverse in the tradition of gopi-Krishna worship, wherein all humans are considered to be "female" *gopis* (cowherd girls) longing for the Male-Beyond-Male Deity, Lord Krishna. While traveling in India, I came across a small band of such *sari*-dressed, smilingly shy, and cosmetically beautified gopis, living beyond any scientia categories of "males who cross-dress as females."

4
Purposeful Urdhvaretas

Urdhvaretas yoga can be approached from many life situations—whether you are partnered or single, caring for children or elders or not—and there are many possible reasons to take up its ways. Perhaps you are intently looking for or merely "open to meeting" someone who will send you flying into the love zone (and vice versa), but the current sex-on-first-date scene has shown you its limitations. Or perhaps you want to mature the urdhvaretic-entheogenic body with a lifelong love-mate. Or as a childless yoga-centered single person, you may be drawn to the advanced realms of the inner marriage of the legendary yogis. Or as an elder with grandchildren and even great-grandchildren, who is beginning to see "the other shore," you are inspired by the "letting go" aspect of a yoga-centered life.

Whatever your life situation or reason, the insights and practices detailed in later chapters of this book—which include guidance in meditation (chapter 5), communication (chapters 8 and 9), relational worship (chapter 10), and hatha yoga (chapter 11)—will nurture your urdhvaretic unfoldment. In fact, all of the hundreds, if not thousands, of yoga practices are, inherently, a manifestation and cultivator of urdhvaretas.

WHO CHOOSES URDHVARETAS?

Here are some vignettes of all sorts of people taking up the worldview and practices of ars erotica urdhvaretas for a variety of reasons. But like having a child or going to a first yoga class for certain reasons, matters can soon get much vaster and more profound.

Ed and Marcie had been on other sexual adventures together, enacting favorite fantasies and going away for frequent romantic weekends alone or with polyamorous communities or yearly Burning Man bacchanalias. One day Ed had a more curious idea and asked Marcie how it would be if they built up their desire for each other for two or so months before expressing it sexually. Four months of being exquisitely attracted to each other went by before they made love, once, and then returned to their "building up time." Then they discovered tantric brahmacharya; when they began to practice sunrise yogic worship they began to experience blossoming feelings in their spines and all their cells a-tingle, all of which fitted naturally into their new "nonsexual" rhythm. They especially liked hours and hours of Nyasa (see chapter 10, page 180), the intercourse of anointing the midbrow pathways in each other till the bursts of light would come and set each other aglow with "warm honey,"* as they called "that inner-sunrise *moment, that* blooming point of no return." Somehow their goal of sex after some months of "buildup" just went away for a year in the midst of dawn wonders and "tango-cognac yoga" (as they uniquely named their yoga worship). Then a dream came to Marcie about orphan adoption that she told Ed about. Without missing a beat, looking straight at each other, both of them beamed even brighter and immediately said, "*Yes* . . . let's do it!"

Sergey, sixteen, went to a yoga retreat with his mother and heard how a chosen period of yogic celibacy known as brahmacharya can contribute to one's personal development. He liked yoga and meditation, so he decided to try it. He also believed the yoga books he read that stated that brahmacharya had been the core of all yoga and

---

*Such inner honey is known as *madhu* in yogic terms, and from it the honey wine known as mead got its name.

yogic enlightenments for thousands of years for millions of yogis and Buddhist saints, as articulated by The Mother, the lifelong spiritual consort of Sri Aurobindo who first described an "Integral Yoga":

> What was the secret of that gigantic intellectuality, spirituality and superhuman moral force which we see pulsating in . . . the ancient philosophy [of yoga] . . . supreme poetry, art, sculpture and architecture? . . . We shall find the secret . . . in a profound knowledge of human psychology and its subtle application to the methods of intellectual training and instruction . . . the all-important discipline of Brahmacharya.[1]

Sergey said he was ready for "the big leagues of yoga" instead of the studio yoga that seemed like "souped-up fitness classes" to him. He was rebellious and wanted the "real thing." His yoga teacher, Natalia, found out; always open to learning from her students, she became inspired, and now hosts a mystical circle kirtan group to celebrate and grow together as inner-married yogis. And yes, this is in Russia.

Mary was fed up with dating, with not being called back the next day, and with how much sex had come to rule her life. IUDs, the Pill, and abortion left her feeling uneasy. Tantric brahmacharya gave her a positive way out of her withdrawal, and yoga classes brought new friendships. She regained her openness, threw out her contraceptives, and feels good about her choices. The yoga practices reconnected her with her fertile womanhood, as well as her flexibility. When the base of her spine came alive with quiet tingles, she called me at the Kundalini Clinic. "Yes, Mary, that is the very first stirrings of Divine Mother Kundalini, called *pranotthana,* and it is like a pregnancy or a puberty." Her sexuality was getting liberated from the compromising ways of scientia sexualis, and the depths of urdhvaretas were expanding within her.

Father Tom found that yoga asanas and breathing exercises helped balance his bodily energies and thus supported his priestly vow of celibacy. He felt less distracted, and his daily prayer life deepened. He told a few of his friends, who then joined him in what they called "Christian Yoga," which led to small contemplative retreats in monastic settings.

During his session with me at the Kundalini Clinic, he wondered whether hundreds, if not thousands, of priests, nuns, and monastics could deepen their spiritual lives through this Christian Yoga. A similar but nascent curiosity manifested when I met with a glowing, beard-flowing Orthodox monk in a small village in Russia. He was reading the Russian edition of *Eros, Consciousness, and Kundalini* as we parted that day.

Jan was so afraid of the health hazards of sex that she overreacted; tantric brahmacharya was merely a strategy to make her abstinence easier. Then she started having some unexpected beneficial experiences in her yoga practice. Tim was impressed, and they started going out together. Their brahmacharya now has nothing to do with safe sex; it has a life of its own. They arise at 5 am together for solo yoga practices, followed by a few partnered poses, and are discovering how spontaneous asanas really are living tumescences of ars erotica. Their relational worship practices, described in chapter 10, have also "come alive," sometimes with tears of closeness and other times with hysterical laughter at the "secret of no-sex liberation" that they have discovered. As old hippies, they often had Jefferson Airplane's song "Share a Little Joke" playing in the background at such "hyena orgasm moments," with its lyric, "Sounded like he'd make a halo, when I heard his laughter floating . . . He said he just let go."[2]

Melanie and Renee had "sexual issues." Just touching fingertips was all they felt comfortable with when I first met them as clients in couples' therapy. But when they touched this way, sitting across from one another, tears would flow, followed by a long embrace. I left the session room to give them privacy. They were discovering a natural brahmacharya of their own hearts' longings. After some months of sessions, they had explored Nyasa and other relational worship sharings of their own creation. Months later they told me of having shared some moments of the Sringara realm of chapter 12.

Lisa had been teaching yoga for five years. Her awakening came while chanting kirtan with her students. "Tears of joy" was the only descriptive phrase that made any sense to her. Her whole life was transformed. She went to India, found a guru at his distant hermitage, reached only by crossing several creeks, and received his shaktipat initiation, took a lifelong brahmacharya vow, and returned some months later to her hometown to open a yoga studio, "The Inner-Mounting Flame." Yes, she was also a fan of the legendary East-West fusion band, Mahavishnu Orchestra.

What brings a person to consider brahmacharya, in any of its various forms—a broken romance, a penchant to be different, a search for something deeper, being tired of the sexual merry-go-round, yoga class experiences, reading about Buddha's inner marriage nirvana, confounding sexual issues, curiosity, fate—cannot be easily explained. In erotic matters, we always are entering a mystery, and often we only discover afterward the real reasons we got involved. In a yogic cosmology, which includes reincarnation, one might find out only a *long* time afterward. According to the theory of karma, our psyches are literally reborn from the seeds of our inner motives, stirring us to live them out in the next moment (or in the next lifetime); this is how the mystery of our relationships develops its circuitous plot.

WHY YOU MIGHT CHOOSE BRAHMACHARYA

YOU ARE GOING TO BE INVOLVED IN A PROJECT FOR SOME TIME, AND YOU THINK TANTRIC BRAHMACHARYA WILL HELP YOU TO FOCUS YOUR TIME AND ENERGY.

Celibacy has long been part of certain traditional lifestyles of service and personal development. Mother Teresa, Mahatma Gandhi, and United Nations Secretary-General Dag Hammarskjöld are three well-known exemplars of choosing celibacy as a support to work and service. Research conducted by Gabrielle Brown, author of *The New Celibacy,* attests to a correlation between unusually creative people and celibacy.

The principles of *karma yoga,* the yoga of life activities, might be particularly relevant to a period of brahmacharya yoga practice that serves a creative project or activity: to enjoy the process of your work at each step, rather than focusing too much on the gratification of completion. Meditation becomes particularly useful in conjunction with brahmacharya for a creative project. When the mind becomes still in meditation, currents of energy begin to flow up through very subtle pathways, invigorating consciousness and inspiring new visions and ideas. We also become freer from personal desires and more objective in our perceptions and assessments. Indeed, you might start brahmacharya to focus your energies on a desired project goal and end up over the years and decades unlocking the retas Source realm of all incarnations: this is the mystery.

YOU ARE FEELING SECLUSIVE.

As one of my teachers used to say, urdhvaretas yoga is discovering the love in yourself that you usually reserve for falling in love with someone else. She claimed it was an ideal preparation for a relationship or a satisfying lifestyle in itself, based on discovering one's inner source of happiness.

Meditative peace is itself an inner form of being alone, for we are free of that crowd of chattering thoughts that can endlessly distract us. Such inner quiet holds the possibility of discovering a profound paradox: we are each singularly alone in the world, yet, in this undistracted silence, we feel even more intimately related to one another and to the world. If you are single, you might choose to use your personal time to practice three or four hours of yoga almost daily, while enjoyably and responsibly maintaining your other involvements. For some single brahmacharins, *sadhana* might become "the love of your life"—at least for the months or years or decades of your practice. Indeed, in India, yogis would take *vrata* "vows" for thousands of lifetimes!

YOU HAVE A SEXUALLY COMMUNICABLE DISEASE, AND YOU WANT SAFE WAYS TO EXPRESS LOVE, PASSION, AND AFFECTION.

HIV, herpes, chlamydia, and other sexually transmitted diseases are demarcating the limits of a territory that earlier sexologists depicted as an idyllic paradise. You might be feeling unjustly backed into this seemingly claustrophobic corner of "no sex" for longer than you expected. Tantric brahmacharya will reveal many alluring gateways out of that boxed-in place.

YOU WANT TO DEVELOP NONSEXUAL FRIENDSHIPS, AND YOU ARE BEING MORE SELECTIVE THESE DAYS.

We are used to seeing one another either as possible sexual partners or as "just friends" (that is, "There is no way I could be turned on to you!"). An inner yes/no switch automatically catalogs everyone we see as sexually desirable or undesirable. In tantric brahmacharya, we can operate beyond this binary narrowness via the unprepared openness of "nonattachment."

Though nonattachment may sound austere, it simply refers to an experience of intimacy without scientia sexualis agendas. We learn to see others without appropriating or grasping at them for some desired end. Our attractions to others often take on a freeing and relaxed intimacy when the expectation of sex has been put aside.

YOU WANT TO DEVELOP A DEEPENING SENSE OF INTIMACY WITH YOUR PARTNER.

Intimacy is a matter of one person being moved by another. The sultry rustle of her robe, the glowing shyness of his gratitude, the heat of her disappointed hopefulness, the anguish of his love-shredding grief, even possessions can be mediums through which we are moved by one another. For it is not the "things" that move us but the way our love brings them to life with the individuality of the beloved. In Saint-Exupéry's *The Little Prince,* the fox speaks of such intimacy, which he calls "taming":

> If you tame me, it will be as if the sun came to shine in my life. I shall know the sound of a step that will be different from all others. . . . And then look: you see the grain-fields down yonder? I do not eat bread. Wheat is of no use to me. The wheat fields have nothing to say to me. And that is sad. But you have hair that is the color of gold. Think how wonderful that will be when you have tamed me! The grain, which is golden, will bring me back the thought of you. And I shall love to listen to the wind in the wheat. . . .
>
> The fox gazed at the little prince, for a long time.
>
> "Please—tame me!" he said.[3]

So often, however, the impatient desire for more intimacy is what obscures the subtle phenomena of intimacy presently alive, as, sadly, the little prince responded to his fox:

"I want to [tame you], very much," the little prince replied. "But I have not much time. I have friends to discover, and a great many things to understand."[4]

To which the fox responded in parting:

"And now here is my secret, a very simple secret: It is only with the heart that one can see rightly; what is essential is invisible to the eye."[5]

YOU ARE TROUBLED BY THE DIFFICULTIES IN LOVE RELATIONSHIPS AND WONDER HOW URDHVARETAS PRACTICES AND SPIRITUAL PSYCHOLOGY MIGHT HELP.

If you are not currently in a love relationship, the practice of solitary brahmacharya can give your life a satisfying fullness of emotionality, commitment, and passion typically thought available only to coupled people. Thus, your longings for a partner can be freed of the desperation that being alone sometimes breeds. Instead, should you meet someone you are truly interested in, your longings will have a welcoming freshness.

Tantric brahmacharya is far more paradoxical and poetic than most conventional and popular psychologies of love. Instead of a vocabulary of black and white, semidiagnostic terms, such as codependency, emotional wounding, or fears of abandonment and commitment, bhakti terms such as *viyoga*—the union that lives quaveringly as longing, hope, or faith, particularly during the most painful struggles—grasp the ambiguity inherent in erotic difficulties. At such times, some people find God, because they feel, now, they *really* need God.

Thus, you will learn about the hidden rectifying powers within apology and forgiveness, how to miss someone romantically instead of thinking of yourself as abandoned, how to protect "the awe of great possibilities" from being misinterpreted as fears of commitment. Fear and awe are close cousins in erotic matters, and it is an ironic tragedy that the same *awesomeness* that inspires feelings of total possibilities in the beginning of love and family life will claustrophobically close down possibilities when misunderstood or merely "labeled" as *fear*. Take a look: are there any substantive dangers? A "danger" of "getting repressed," perhaps? Or perhaps it is only Dr. Freud's *scientia sexualis* boilerplate that is getting you to think such worries into your consciousness.

In the ars erotica of faith and uncertainty, far beyond psychology's medical model of "where do I hurt?" we encounter the paradoxical and lesser-known erotic passions of joys that seem too good to be true, of ourselves or our parents and partners being more than we ever thought, even as we awaken to other possibilities that seem too tragic to be endured. We uncover the too common irony that sometimes it becomes easier to fight over personality issues and mundane problems than to get all choked up with one's gratitude. We spare each other our gratitudes, for the ensuing intimacy and bonding is more than we can readily bear.

YOU WONDER IF YOUR MARRIAGE CAN BE ENHANCED IN CERTAIN WAYS BY A TIME OF REGULAR COUPLE AND SOLO YOGA PRACTICES.

Marriage exists because we need the time of a lifetime to bring forth more completely the deeply hidden potentialities that begin to emerge when people are in love with each other. Commitment is merely the natural and immediate response to perceived, yet hidden, possibilities. Commitment is the sustained and suspenseful allurement of mystery.

Practicing partner yoga in the spirit of ars erotica allows couples to share so much vitality and intimacy that they are just as rewarded by an hour of such shared practice as they would be in lovemaking. After two months of such a switch, the vitality, closeness, and energetic awakenings could very likely be even more persuasive and after six months or a year or two or ten, even more "entheogenically" persuasive. Then, like Robert Frost, they might feel:

Two roads diverged in a wood, and I—
I took the one less traveled by,
And that has made all the difference.

YOU FIND THE VARIOUS ARTIFICIAL METHODS OF CONTRACEPTION TO BE UNDESIRABLE, AND YOU WONDER IF THERE ARE "OTHER WAYS" TO MAKE LOVE.

When Wilhelm Reich was formulating his basic principles of sexual liberation for fertile heterosexuals, he concluded that, since sex was necessary thrice weekly, contraception was "absolutely necessary for sexual health." Within the conventional biological model of sex, this may be true. Yet this solution is not as utopian as Reich and the rest of us had hoped—as our abortion rates and problems with contraception can attest.

Contraception, unintended pregnancy, abortion, and the debates surrounding them, are rendered obsolete for the tantric brahmacharin, just as they are in the fully matured stages of urdhvaretas, when male-female shared eroticism becomes so devotional that all the rasas of fertility transform into entheogenic internal secretions and the pariyanga of endless eroticism. Before such maturity arrives in the shared-gender mystery of gradual brahmacharya, contraceptives—understood as training wheels, more than as "protections against unwanted pregnancies"—*are clearly in order.*

Feeling the daring profundity of life creation as awe and wonder, not mere unwanted fertility or even "wanted" fertility, is also crucial to gaining golden experience of what life is, what there is "beyond our de-seeded egoic desires," and what a male, a woman, a child, a zygote is. Having intercourse only when hoping to conceive can help us recover the actual *experience* of procreation. Rob, forty, describes his surprise of "discovering" that sex is also the procreative process:

After several years of seed-enhancing, urdhvaretas yoga, it was easy to feel the procreative aspect of sex. When we did conceive, it was one of the most profound experiences of my life. I had lost all my sexual associations with the act of intercourse, and all that I was aware of were the sensations of conceiving this unique, new human being with my wife.

On one hand I was amazed—this is a miracle! On the other hand I felt convinced—so this is what sex is about. I could see why some religions have tried to keep sex just for reproduction, although I doubt they had this sort of experience in mind. It felt so real, so meaningful, that it has changed my understanding of what human life is all about, of how much spiritual power we have as human beings.

The sublimative way of erotic expression could also be particularly useful to teenagers, whose sexual curiosity forever outsmarts even the most well-schooled efforts of our sex/contraception education. Originally, the term brahmacharya referred to preadolescence through young adulthood, when, in the wake of genital puberty, we learn and grow at a rapid pace. An open-minded teenager might find brahmacharya very fulfilling, rather than being one more nagging parental injunction against which to rebel. (In support of this, please see the section in chapter 7 entitled "Ars Erotica Facts of Life for Teenagers").

YOU HAVE BEEN CELIBATE FOR SOME TIME NOW, AND YOU ARE WONDERING WHAT MIGHT BE GOING ON IN YOU AS A RESULT.

Having a vocabulary to apply to your brahmacharya experiences can be most helpful, especially in a culture where any lifestyle without sex could be understood as an absence of erotic experiences. If you have been practicing any form of spiritual celibacy for some time, the mere publication of this book may be important to you.

There is no "one size fits all" urdhvaretas. I hope I was able to tap into a few of your individual and particular reasons for considering brahmacharya. Other answers to the question of why you would choose it for a time or forever might come from something that stirs deep within you. Your urdhvaretas yoga might be helpfully understood most fundamentally as a continuation of the retas mystery from whence you incarnated and were born. You might want to meditate on the "Retas Mysteries" meditation in chapter 7 to explore those depths. Likewise, the rest of this book might reveal some reasons you did not know you could even *have*.

BEGINNING
AND SETTING A TIME FRAME

If you decide to try purposeful urdhvaretas, I recommend you set a minimum duration of three months "without sex or masturbation or hot movies." As moralistic as this sounds, it won't remain that way, as ars erotica experiences will come to allure you, "seduce" you, thrill and transfix you in both utter tranquility and uplifting energy. You need some time to reorient yourself to the ars erotica perspective within the everyday world of sexual attraction. It will take some time for you to truly engage with the choice that you have made and to reap the results of greater tolerance for having what you used to call "sexual feelings" without thinking you must act on "them" in conventional ways. Indeed, you will soon see that all such feelings come to us without name tags. Then you might find yourself just "letting go."

You may or may not find a great deal of anxiety in setting the duration of your practice. Should a period of more than a few months shock you, I would advise you to think again about what you want and what you believe about your sexual situation. Urdhvaretas is more than a weekend workshop or another "style" of yoga. It requires a sincere and devoted application of oneself to develop its potentials.

Through the energy-transfer initiation (*diksha*) known as shaktipat, the yogic transformations described in this book can be given a strong jump start. Here the role of the trusted teacher or guru must be considered. Although the reputations of certain spiritual teachers have been marred in recent times, studying with a respected guru and receiving his or her energetic initiation—via a mantra, touch, eye contact, or other means—can prove invaluable. The experience, love, and support of such a person can add so much inspiration to one's life and practice that gratitude of the highest order often emerges. All the technical knowledge and long-sought attainments can pale in comparison with such feelings. Yet the guru desires our growth, so the thanks he or she prefers is our dedication to these ways of living.

If you can find a shaktipat yoga guru in the United States to initiate your brahmacharya, that would be exceptional, since most such advanced yogis are in India, though typically hidden from yoga tourism's view. Without a shaktipat initiatory boost, perhaps your gains will be slower. But perhaps inspirations and "boosts" will come to you in myriad other ways, such as dreams, woodland walks, art-creation moments, or while being moved by sacred chanting.

My first commitment was for fifteen months. After that, I had a one-time sexual liaison, went "hmmm" to myself, and immediately resumed my ars erotica yoga. Thereafter, I stopped counting and thus added another dimension to my practice, an almost frightening sense of freedom. Initially, ambivalent feelings took the form of the thought, "When is this going to be over?" But romantic song lines such as, "There ain't no mountain high enough" inspired me to continue, along with myriad inner and outer experiences.[6] That gives rise to another question for you to consider: if you (as an individual or a couple) really start to have profound experiences and sustaining inspirations in the months ahead, on what basis would you decide to stop?

You might insist that you'll know exactly when to return to conventional sex. Ramakrishna, an Indian saint who went deeply into the practice of brahmacharya, described his experience as "one in which it seemed that all the pores of the skin were like female organs and intercourse was taking place over the whole body." Such experiences, which may emerge only after years of development, can make the decision to stop or continue far more thought-provoking than those within the folds of scientia sexualis might imagine. Scientia Church celibates will also have a challenge, though "the inner embraces of the Divine" are part of their charismatic mysticisms as well. Dance your inner embraces with the Divine or dance with dancing itself! Sing with singing itself, and enter the kingdom within!

Not setting a specific duration can help make your practice less self-conscious and studied. You might even begin to feel a sense of freedom in having no predetermined limit. On the other hand, if you have trouble establishing yourself in your commitment, a preset duration could give you support to pull yourself through the first months of practice and uncertainty.

CONSIDERATIONS OF
PERSONALITY AND MYSTERY

Another formidable consideration is how tantric brahmacharya fits into the idiosyncrasies of your personality. Are you a perfectionist, expecting to get it right the very first time and more and more right as you go along? Or are you spiritually competitive and think brahmacharya will make you "more spiritual" than others? Are you from an older school of sex and feel that abstinence is a proper way to restrain waywardness? Do you tend to go to extremes, expecting to swing from brahmacharya to utter sexual abandon?

Perhaps you consider yourself overly dependent and feel you might be doing this to win someone's approval. Consider whether you might not be trying to avoid the challenges of social interaction by going celibate. Not only is such uneven growth unsatisfying; the high degree of intimacy that tantric brahmacharya works toward will not allow it. Another possibility is that you may be angry at someone and want to inflict your brahmacharya on them as revenge. As you might guess, all such motivations can narrow your yogic experience, at least initially. As you progress, however, more positive motivations based in your new experiences might arise.

If you intend to practice with a partner, observe the manner in which any problems you ordinarily have while talking about sex emerge during your conversations on urdhvaretas tantra. Notice which partner wants to practice it more, who acts as though he or she knows more about it, who is taking it more seriously, and so forth. By returning to the foundation of eros-as-mystery, you will be aided in dislodging yourself from these hierarchical and polarizing dynamics.

Finally, you may be concerned about HIV, problematic relationships, being rejected or getting committed or about sexual performance. It is important that you be as honest as you can about such concerns as you set out on your path. Your brahmacharya practice might even help resolve some of these nagging boilerplate worries of the ego-mind and scientia sexualis psychology as you discover moments of the self-acceptance known as "the peace that passeth all understanding."

You may start out facing the mystery in the form of the question: "Will I experience anything new, or just feel repressed?" Indeed, upswings of retas hormones are not uncommon and might uplift your passions as well. But in purposeful urdhvaretas these ars erotica passions can wonderfully animate asanas, esoteric dancing, kirtan, and the rest. When you break through scientia sexualis, carrying all your freed-up passions with you—what Rumi called one's "tail-feathers"—onto the terra firma of ars erotica expression, well, I can already hear "your laughter floating" as you share "a little joke" with the *shamanica medhra* ecstatic yoga cults of the past five thousand years. Om Shiva!

5
Yogic Anatomy and Transformation of the Ars Erotica Body

Through exceedingly detailed meditations over thousands of hours, ancient yogis determined that the human body is far more than a configuration of fleshy organs, bones, and fluids. They discovered a system of seven *chakras,* or energy regulatory centers, located approximately along the spinal axis. We are also composed of five gradients or *koshas,* literally, "sheaths," each one more interior and subtle than the previous one; thus we are the actual bridge from the physical to the spiritual.

THE SUBTLE BODIES

The sheaths, which are also referred to as "bodies," range from less dense to more dense. Each exerts a guiding intelligence over the next in the following order, starting with the individual soul (jiva): the causal body (*ananda-maya kosha*), the reflective-intellectual body (*vijnana-maya kosha*), mental-emotional body (*mano-maya kosha*), vital energy body (*prana-maya kosha*), and the physical body (*anna-maya kosha*). Through this anatomy of increasingly interior bodies, yoga maps the emotionality and sentient capacities of the intimus itself and thus the way toward deepening our intimacy with one another and the world.

The physical (anna-maya) and vital energy (prana-maya) sheaths operate together, forming the densest of our dimensions, the biological body. The erotic phenomena of sheer sensation, physical-emotional warmth, the various orgasmic reflexes, and hormonal rhythms emerge primarily within these two interacting sheaths.

Erotic pleasures and intimacies of the physical and vital bodies operating together constitute the "realm of the senses," the ideal of a pure sensuality. Within the confines and ideals of scientia sexualis they are seen by the church as the perditious path to hell via "temptations of the flesh" and by modern sexual psychology as a path to heavenly delights on earth, recently wrested from the repressive grip of the church.

Within the ars erotica, however, the interaction of the pranic energy body and the anna-maya (literally, "food-eating") body give rise to bodily pleasures and maturities of a different order, which include all the charismatic "manifestations of the spirit in the flesh" as well as the gestation-completing contractions of maternal labor and the egoless incarnating movements of infants. All such manifestations are catalyzed by awakened seed energy creativities that live in prana-maya kosha life-energy body and ananda-maya kosha, the God-Source of deep nature.

The mental-emotional body (mano-maya kasha) holds the cognitive intelligence by which we identify and attribute a socially agreed-upon meaning to the events and sensations that occur in the two preceding bodies. People who thought they were going to "just have sex" who later feel emotionally involved with their sexual partner have aroused this more intimate sheath during the otherwise seemingly casual sex. Here is where fantasies, desires, joys, jealousies, emotional wounds, angers, hopes, and sorrows reside to be shared with, and hopefully healed by, those whom (or Whom) we trust. This is the realm of placebo cures and psychosomatic illness and faith healing that grows in its power as the still-subtler bodies become involved, too.

This is also the realm where students of meditative still-sitting and yogic pose-holding—whose instructors hold limited or restrictive views of the paths of "being moved"—will be guided to "let the stress-releasing movements pass" without much ars erotica explanation of such tumescences. Cynical certainties and demystified certainties also rumble around here. That means the mental-emotional mind is swayable both by "misery loves company" and by popular spiritual group-mind and galacto-memes. Galacto-memes have their uplifting sweet spots, but then what?

This is where the reflective-intellectual sheath (vijnana-maya kosha) can come to our aid with its overarching powers of refined discernment, informed choice, and innovative creativity. It takes the erotic sentiments, experiences, and interpreted meanings of the mental body one step further. This is the realm of the "Higher Power" of twelve-step-programs. It is where we "learn from experience, or not." Here we empathically grasp the sacred creativity and beauty of the other, so that his or her emotions and thoughts, as well as our own as "inner beauty," come ever more into our evaluations of self and others.

Thus, vijnana-maya kosha is the domain of human character development that extends the "genital primacy ego" toward ars erotica maturity, where ego and superego become a caring team. As Einstein said regarding the towering vijnana genius, Mahatma Gandhi, "Generations to come, it may well be, will scarce believe that such a man as this one ever in flesh and blood walked upon this Earth." Vijnana genius also inspired Nelson Mandela, just released from twenty-seven years of incarceration, to tell stunned government officials who had imprisoned him that he forgave them for their decades of injustices of apartheid.

The reflective-intellectual sheath provides the longer-lasting erotic pleasures and intimacies of loving admiration, the feelings of sincerity and respect, lifelong nurturance and commitment, the romanticisms of love, gratitude, apology, and forgiveness. Here is where we choose to be guided by "higher principles" more than by the exciting immediacies of "beyond judgment" one-night stands. Are we "taking better care of ourselves" or "repressing ourselves" at such times? As Ernest Hemingway put it, "What is moral is what you feel good [about] after, and what is immoral is what you feel bad [about] after." The reflective intellect tries to sift through such boilerplate aphorisms to help us make our final and nuanced assessment, always open to learning more, yet able to feel the finitude of time passage and make "best possible" decisions.

Here, the real enlightenments of wisdom get to the core of many spiritual platitudes beyond their meme versions such as "Be Here Now" or "Follow Your Bliss." Thus, when Ram Dass found out he was a father and grandfather and that family love and "soul love" were "not that different," he openly shared his new wisdom with his followers, rather than burying it. His DNA paternity test gave him real retas wisdom that originates from the ananda-maya kosha and filters into the vijnana-maya kosha regarding the Holy Family that *every* family is, along with the recognition that embodied life manifests as a divine miracle through the seed-activating love that "makes the whole world go around." Such has been the concern of all spiritual traditions wherein the fertility of life itself has remained paramount, for millennia.*

Wisdom, *vidya* in Sanskrit, is matured enlightenment of all the subtle bodies, far more rich and complex than deseeded teachings such as those focusing on the "Power of Now," which tell us to let go of our "assessing minds" (vijnana-maya kosha) while failing to highlight the profundity of the retas connections of all the bodies to the ananda-maya kosha, the underlying causal or bliss body, the most intimate abode of the individual soul, jiva, or *atman*.

Through knowing ananda-maya kosha, semen, ova, and all so-called "sexual hormones" and "reproductive processes" are renamed as "entheogenic rasas" and "procreative wisdom powers." At the causal level, even infertile persons are retas-creating beings; there, each person is a com-

---

*I wince to reconsider the work of a beautiful man who has inspired millions. Yet if Ram Dass (from his spiritually awake state) and his son's mother had raised their son together on a daily, real-life basis, he might then have—for two generations, by this time—been teaching how "soul love" and personal and parental love are "not mutually exclusive" of one another. Instead, he (along with childless Ken Wilber and others whose work has focused on "[solo] spiritual heroes") unwittingly garbled into Western lives the specialized family-less, "no ties" life of the tiny minority—"the *sadhu* trip"—despite the warning against this given by his one-time *sadhu-yoga* mentor, Baba Hari Dass (see Dass, *Silence Speaks*). In this revised history, "spiritual emergence" might include such spiritually challenging moments as those following a positive (or negative) pregnancy test, or the DNA test that profoundly revised Ram Dass's understanding of "soul love." Indeed, the emotional upheaval of possible divorces involving young children might also be viewed as "spiritual emergencies," not just the LSD-like mystical ones of transpersonal interest thus far.

plete being; thus even miraculous physical healings are within its powers. Going into the depths of ananda-maya can help East-West, integral, and transpersonal institutions of cross-cultural transmission to retrue themselves to their sacred mission in the public trust, beyond the sixties effervescence. Similarly, meditation centers and yoga studios and teachers filled with retas-awakened energies can be uplifted toward ars erotica wholeness.

Located in an etheric space within the heart, the bliss body is in intimate rapport with *brahmarandhra,* the subtle center of mind and intellect. Together and in balance, they manifest what the great Dutch philosopher Baruch Spinoza called "the intellectual love of God," thought and love combined.

In ananda-maya kosha, erotic pleasure is permanent, and, independent of efforts or stimulations, it feels "miraculous." Fulfillment in knowing the Source in the causal body can be so great that complete dispassion or nonattachment to sense objects, desires, and thoughts results. One has attained a profound balancing of both the internal and external realms of "needs" and "needing." As the yogi Vyas Dev says, "This is an indescribable state, beyond the pairs of opposites. . . . This is the highest limit of individual knowledge."[1]

Through "self-ishness," that is, the self's overclinging to experience, the clarity of such knowledge can diminish, imbalance emerges, and the ego-self (known as *ahamkara*) gets confused. Ignoring the wisdom of the reflective mind while giving too much credence to the doubts and rebellions of the mental-emotional body, it thinks and feels itself into a separate identity that is historically limited, and scientia sexualis embedded.

On the other hand, when the resources of all the bodies are functioning in balance and the ego-self is able to grasp its more modest place in relationship to the subtler bodies, sexual (and many other) desires arise like small waves upon the deep retas-wisdom ocean of our being. They do not sway us but slip into our depths, gratifying and maturing us as they germinate the many body-soul powers of mature ars erotica life.

THE CHAKRAS

To effect this balancing of all the bodies, tantra attends to the septenary system of chakras: *muladhara, svadhisthana, manipura, anahata, vishuddha, ajna,* and *sahasrara.* Each chakra also generates a specific locus of longings and pleasures associated with its particular properties. Through them we can map the transformations of passion and consciousness from bodily maintenance and survival to divine rapture.

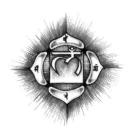

Muladhara Chakra

The first three chakras are associated with the physical body. The first of these, muladhara, the root chakra at the base of the spine, holds the power of fundamental survival and the primal erotic passion to live. Its element is earth. It is closely related to the adrenal glands and is attuned to our instinctive survival needs. In meditation it appears as an earthy, ruddy, red glow.

Concerned with elimination, muladhara has a gutsy feel and a strength that is "not afraid to get its hands dirty." Dependable and earthy, it might be considered the "Ernest Hemingway" of the chakras. Concerned also with the sense of smell, muladhara's instinctive powers can, literally, "smell" trouble, truth, or deception; it is the source of the proverbial nose for news. Pheromones, of course, are biology's name for the way the shared-gender mystery affects muladhara.

At the more esoteric level, the wise "serpent power" called kundalini rests coiled within muladhara, as a residue of the primeval force responsible for guiding embryological gestation as well as the creation of the physical universe. It can be aroused by yogic or other spiritual practices to enter a subtle channel in the spine (*sushumna*), causing a blissful tumescence throughout all the bodies and inspiring a deep sense of reverence and humility. Gopi Krishna, author of *Kundalini: The*

Evolutionary Energy in Man, maintains that all forms of genius involve some degree of awakening of this essence of revelatory intelligence.

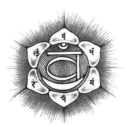

Svadhisthana Chakra

Svadhisthana chakra is located a few inches above the root chakra in the general area of pelvic genital arousal. Its element is water. It is associated with the endless seeds within seeds for all future incarnations and, when disconnected from the life-creating powers of fertility, is the primary basis of conventional sexuality.

Svadhisthana also governs taste and the world of "good taste," which displays itself in fashions as the play of taste and sensuality. Raunchy, sexy, alluring, classic, monastically robed—all are manifestations of svadhisthana, via dress. "Juicy" people with a kind of "chemistry" also reveal something about this chakra but only suggestively so, for that is the manner of svadhisthana. Erotic fantasies and scenarios, as internal adult entertainments, are also stirred in this center by scientia imagery. Thus we might say it is the "Elvis" and "Marilyn" of the chakras. When all the chakras mature via the spinal puberties, ars erotica imagery makes perfect sense, inclusive of Sringara Rasa, grihastha, pariyanga, and saintly solo brahmacharya.

Manipura Chakra

Manipura chakra, the solar plexus center, is where the fire element presides. The whole gamut of heated emotions of jealousy, anger, vanity, belly laughter, and willful assertiveness is based here. Manipura is associated with the navel, and feelings of dependency and autonomy relate to it, as well as the psychological ideal of "emotional honesty." When matured with all the chakras, spiritually attuned sentiments uplift us ever more into the emotional honesties such as love, compassion, and forgiveness.

As the most elevated of the three physical body chakras, this is the site of existential struggles to believe in "higher realities." The loss of "groundedness" can also happen in manipura via the "flight to the light," or "flakiness" phenomenon, whereby a thin veneer of spiritual development is mistaken for a more mature attainment. Ken Wilber has referred to this foible as the "pre-transpersonal fallacy." To achieve spiritual growth, one needs to have gutsiness, juice, and "stomach," as well as heart and soul and the wisdom of life experience. Perhaps Amelia Earhart, Fritz Perls, and C. Everett Koop are manipura types.

Manipura holds critical importance in urdhvaretas, where retas is matured by the heat of this solar center into ojas, a nonphysical constituent in the radiance of consciousness. The beauty of this radiance also allures kundalini to rise from muladhara.

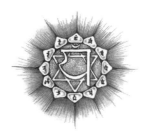

Anahata Chakra

Anahata chakra, the heart center, is related to the air element. Here the language of emotional needs is replaced by that of devotional needs, which is to say, "I need" has become "I love" or "I feel devotional yearnings." The soul is reaching beyond the ego's hopes for self-directed autonomy and emotional closeness and senses the fulfillments of a shared reality. Indeed, the limited sense of the separate-self ego comes to light.

The soul abides in anahata, the heart chakra, with its finer sensitivities and courage (from *couer,* "heart"), which often exceed good sense and sensual familiarities. Sustained by the gutsiness of muladhara, the daring of svadhisthana, and the willingness of manipura, anahata can become inspired. In anahata, compassion opens toward "there but for the grace of God go I." Love shows us that the happiness of the other is our happiness and the mystery of giving is like receiving, or better. Thus, we face various contradictions among value systems in moving from the first three chakras, which oversee the physical body, to the heart, the first chakra that governs supraphysical resources and realms of erotic meaning.

When we feel love for someone attractive to us, anahata and svadhisthana can both be stirred, and we can feel pulled in two directions, one familiar and lush, the other more mysterious and distant feeling. To continue in tantric urdhvaretas maturation at such times, we must let go of the seeming certainty that the heat of sex would be so *right* with this person we love. Instead, we must take the leap of faith into the millennia of ars erotica teachings. Through such faith, ojas intensifies and entheogenic awakenings can occur, as we see with Lianne and Andy.

Lianne had been observing brahmacharya and engaging in meditation and devotional practices in a yoga community for five years when she met Andy. He moved into the community mainly to be near Lianne but was interested enough in yoga to take on the various practices. During the first year their friendship grew and so did Andy's understanding of urdhvaretas. They saw each other primarily in larger group settings. Lianne was moved by Andy's dedication, and during the second year of his residency she was falling more in love with him. On one of their morning walks Andy reached out to Lianne.

The moment of awkwardness lasted about one second and they embraced. All of a sudden it was as though she had never lived urdhvaretically; she felt like a "teenager in love." A rapid succession of sexual images raced through her mind. She hoped that they would surrender to this passion and at the same time hoped that they wouldn't. Andy thought that after two years, they were finally together, but he, too, was of two minds, not knowing where his feelings would lead him.

As their embrace continued, first Lianne, then Andy, started to laugh. It was so funny thinking about how impossible it was to know what to do with each other. Their embrace took on the warmth of a shared, unexpected discovery. They were still laughing when they kissed each other and fell down together.

As they looked up, the sky and the air everywhere seemed pink. The trees seemed to be visibly breathing, in a kind of oceanic harmony with their breaths. It was as if their love had carried them to some hidden space where even the air was alive with love and magic. They were there together and had preserved the essence of their yogic passion.

Such ars erotica discoveries on the brink of desire are not unlike the feelings you get when you have approached a deeply inviting pool, seemingly too wide to jump across, but you jump anyway. Through the tantric leap of meditation, conventional images of "hot sexuality" and a pejorative sense of a squelching "abstinence" no longer appear as accurate mappings of the ways of love and erotic freedom. Instead, the images of sex desire can seem to be metaphorical, instead of literal, suggestive of something yet unknown and quite liberating and exquisite.

To get to this new place, we need faith and the entheogenic light of ojas (radiantly glowing bioenergy). But how can we make subtle discernments between gradations of loving passion when frequent sexual activity quickly raises, then dramatically lowers, ojas levels? Virya—perhaps related to oxytocin—precipitates like sweet butter from fine cream. Felt as a catapulting breakthrough that keeps stretching and encompassing more and more, or as a courage that follows the star that myriad yogis and Buddhas have all followed, virya sparkles with virtue. Strategies and plans to "find love" become unimportant. Heartfelt faith prevails, and one who has lived decades of scientia sexualis ways is able to take leaps of faith to the next and the next ars erotica bodily awakenings. While ojas clarifies the more aesthetic subtleties of emotion with its light, virya ignites the compassion of "heart-consciousness."

As a healing side effect, emotional pains mysteriously transform; bitterness and cynicism drop away. The harshly tragic aspects of human life have met their match—compassionate love—and the soul matures the ego-personality through these difficulties. Thus, forbearance, sacrifice, anger without vengeance, courageous action, and, at times, a diverting humor ennoble us and deepen our characters with the softened gnarl of experience. Lord Christ, Albert Schweitzer, Adi Ji Narayan, Mr. Rogers, and perhaps a certain person you know well embody the qualities of anahata chakra.

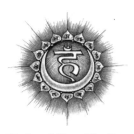

Vishuddha Chakra

The elemental ether that lives in vishuddha is even more subtle than air (the element of the heart). Vishuddha permeates words with their spirit, their near-ineffable meanings, nuances, and innuendos often lost when communications are too literal. Words are "shaped currents of air," thus "the word become flesh" is found as the opened heart. Scientia literalness can be reversed by listening with vishuddha's ars erotica–attuned ear; then the myriad asana "poses" and mudra "symbol-energy-seals" become rasa-infused "tumescences." The meaning of brahmacharya then is released from its endless mistranslation as "celibacy" (a kiss-of-death term) or even "following the Absolute" into, quite simply, "inner marriage."

Sacred chanting can uplift to spontaneous and freely impassioned anahata-nad, whereby the entheogenic elixirs of the rasas soar in the deep ars eroticism of bhakti yoga.* Sufic *qawwali,* Judaic *nigune,* Pentacostal *glossolalia,* Tibetan *gyuto* overtone, and Gregorian modes of sacred chanting all emerge here, too, as ars erotica passions of the voice, each with throbbing, quivering orgasmic reach, often beyond public performance relevance. For thirty years chanting became my brahmacharya lovemaking activity, par excellence, and I can fully attest to its all-night, never-ending passions, delicate call-and-response intricacies, thunderously sweaty spinal crescendos, and playful surprises.

---

*I refer you to my chanting recordings with Axis Mundi that have prompted Silvia Nakkach, Indian vocalist master and thirty-year student of Ali Akbar Khan, to call me "one of the three or four greatest kirtan chanters in the U.S." Why so? The urdhvaretas entheogenic ecstasies of decades of chanting can in no other way be replicated.

God/Goddess names the supreme "Seed of all seeds" powers behind the retas powers of anahata-nad chanting that push the voice beyond entertainment and performance relevance. It is this hyper-reality of an "exceedingly, beyond-human-knowing" God/Goddess Power that has allured saints for millennia into profound inner marriages far beyond scientia credibility and "lazy man's guides to enlightenment." It is this God/Goddess Power that is desperately prayed to, "please, God, please," to avert an impending war "in every pre-battle foxhole, where there are no atheists." In this quote from the Indic "Song of God," vishuddha chakra has tried to put the excessive power of God into words, for the merely human Arjuna to know him. Barely:

> Look, Arjuna: thousands,
> millions of my divine forms,
> of every color and shape.

> Look: the sun gods, the gods
> of fire, dawn, sky, wind, storm,
> wonder that no mortal has ever
> beheld! Look, Arjuna!

> The whole universe, all things,
> animate or inanimate,
> are gathered here—look!—enfolded
> inside my infinite body.

> But since you are not able
> to see me with mortal eyes,
> I will grant you divine sight. Look!
> Look! The depth of my power![2]

This is vishuddha chakra's honor: to channel some of this infinite God Power toward solving problems that are "impossible, until they are done," as Nelson Mandela put it and lived it. When all hope is lost to us because we are in too much pain or fear or, worse, because we are blinded by greed or vengeance, we can pray for help. Yes, seeing the better qualities in someone who has just cheated you or killed your foxhole buddy in the bloodlusts of war is a tall order. Still, the waverings of the heart receive a whispered steadying from the clearer objectivity of vishuddha, quickening the words of the heart with *prema,* unconditioned love, and vishuddha expressive passions.

Indeed, if two camps of enemies *both* leapt to "love thine enemy" vishuddha passions, all history would radically uplift. Thus, King Solomon discerned the baby's true mother from the false when the latter was willing to cut the child in half while the true mother would willingly give up her own child to spare him.

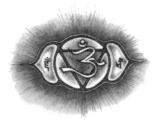

Ajna Chakra

Ajna, "the third eye," is where, as the Bible notes, "thine eyes become single," where there is no longer a difference between male and female, and where "the peace that passeth all understanding" dwells. Erotic mystery persists as the continuous, inexplicable unfolding of creation, maturation, dissolution, and re-creation. Matured wisdom culminates in *vairagha* (nonattachment), the wisdom of enriched objectivity and Divine Power inspirations based in perineum-to-pineal, all-functioning fullness. In such ultra-objectivity, one is capable of the wisest and most nuanced of perceptions and decisions far beyond black-and-white polarizations. Indeed, one can "see" time passing and become intuitively prescient. Ah, real *wisdom*! All the previous chakras can be further refined in their specific sensitivities, altogether creating a great "board of directors" with each contributing its area of wisdom.

Related to the secretion of amrita, the nectar of immortality, ajna awakening (in conjunction with all the chakras) bestows the hypothalamus-pineal puberty, in which a myriad of rasas secrete orgasmic capacities. Indeed, according to neuroendocrinology, the "little wedding chamber" hypothalamus is the origin of numerous secretions and sensations of yearnings and bliss, all known and named by ars erotica traditions.*

Kisses become, literally, "sweeter than wine," via salivary ptyalin that opens up the sweetness of all food, further enriched with salivary immunoglobin A (via glandular chemistry corresponding to feelings of love, admiration, and compassion), which makes each other both delicious and ars erotically intoxicating.† Entwined lovers create higher states via a literal fleshing out of the Marcusian concept of a "spiritualization of the instincts" (see chapter 1, pages 24–25) that physiologically occurs as the hypothalamic "instinct-satiety center" undergoes its secretional puberty from manifesting "desire-satiety" chemistries into manifesting "spiritual longings-bliss" chemistries.‡

---

*I recall my experiments done with hypothalamus world expert, Bartley Hoebel at Princeton, where lab rats would "bar-press" to send electrical stimuli to this "satiety center" over and over, to the point of near-total exhaustion. In gratitude to Dr. Hoebel for his scientia sexualis inspiration of my yogic inner research on "the little wedding chamber," please see www.psychologicalscience.org/index.php/publications/observer/2011/november-11/bartley-g-hoebel.html.

†For details and images on the embryology of tongue-hypothalamus development, when an inner sweetness literally swallows the tongue away from its cranial "heaven realm" contact with the proto-hypothalamus and into the then-forming mouth cavity to serve as the taste center for the earthy, food-eating anna-maya flesh-body, see Sovatsky, *A Phenomenological Exploration of Orgasmic, Tantric and Brahmacharya Sexualities,* 133–35; for the reversal of this process whereby the tongue flips back and reaches away from the food-tasting realm and back into the *akhashic* or heaven realm in khechari "heaven-space" mudra, see Sovatsky, "Kundalini and the Complete Maturation of the Ensouled Body."

‡What Marcuse intuited in 1955 as a remedy for rampant capitalist greed became visible to me in 1970 in those lab rats as they repeatedly awakened pleasure secretions in their hypothalami, and as my own tongue and hypothalamus first quivered in me in 1976 via yogic mysteries of a greed-freeing bliss through shaktipat vibrations from a guru I hadn't even met (see chapter 1, page 18).

Altogether, the powers of *tapas* (the ardor of sustained selfless, heat-purifying passion), *tejas* (electrical brilliance), soma (uplifted, dimethyltryptamine-like visionary experiences), and amrita (rejuvenating and inner-light melatonin awakenings) combine and give rise to auras (the golden, auric glow of matured sainthood, such as that which roused an elder British judge, in spite of himself, to stand up in head-bowed respect for the golden-glowing accused, Mahatma Gandhi, as the latter entered his courtroom).*

Together they manifest every sort of ecstasy: ars erotic plays and joys, entheogenic mind expansions, selfless love, heart-rending unions and gratitude, body-jolting surges. In the full pubescent flow of these rasas, one develops principled character and the wise vision to see virtue hidden (perhaps in convoluted or even deranged and horrific forms) in human acts, everywhere. We become capable of loving our enemies while also liberating them from their twisted anguish and trapped expressions of self-interest, such as when Jimmy Carter's inspired sharing of baby pictures with Anwar Sadat and Menachem Begin provoked a shared, grandfatherly burst of all sorts of retas powers, catapulting them to working out the Camp David Accords, though the treaty, backed with billions of bilaterally spent dollars, has been constantly threatened by skirmishes.†

Beyond the din of despondently cynical or unconvincingly optimistic demystifying opinions and scientia myopic "truths," urdhvaretas brings to life the yogic siddhis or powers noted in myriad sacred texts. One might say to herself, "Oh my! I have become like the actual Buddha!" Or "We have become the mythic Shiva-Shakti couple!"

Certain uncompromising devotees of the penultimate ajna prefer to bypass the many substeps and complexities of tantric

---

*See R. Attenborough's film *Gandhi* for a tear-evoking cinematic portrayal of that moment of "spiritual purity prevailing over societal power."
†I learned of the "baby photo" catalyst in 1979 while casually talking about unreported "spiritual moments in politics" with Hubert Humphrey's speechwriter, Milton Friedman, who was at Camp David at the time. Please see the 2007 documentary *Jimmy Carter, Man from Plains* for President Carter's telling of the story).

brahmacharya that I have described. Following the precepts of traditional monasticism, they attempt, in one leap, to attune to ajna, typically including vishuddha (practice of constant, repetitive prayers to one's deity) and anahata (selfless surrender via service or ecstatic devotion). Couples' practices and even the concept of energetic transformation are dismissed or left unexplored. For some of these devotees, brahmacharya is either easy and spontaneous or a concerted discipline without recourse to any yogic techniques. The call of God, guru, Divine Love, and the sufferings of the world family have uplifted millions of people beyond romantic, nuclear-familial, and material aspects of a "personal life."

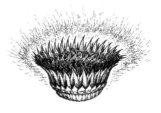

Sahasrara Chakra

The seventh or crown chakra, sahasrara, is of such a spiritual nature that restrictions of time, space, the anna-maya kosha, and even mortality are completely transcended, as in many life-changing near-death experiences. Sahasrara is the thousand-petaled lotus of holy effulgence, experienced as the light of ten million suns; "like mercury light kept in a vessel of silver. The thousands of convolutions of the brain appear like the luminous petals of a lotus," says the inwardly-sighted yogi Vyas Dev. When Thomas Aquinas had such an experience in the year before he died, he called all his previous writing, including the *Summa Theologica*, "straw."

Reverent awe, unremitting joy, and spiritual freedom are the qualities of the mystery in sahasrara. Inner light dazzles the meditator, as described in this passage by Allama Prabhu, in *Speaking of Siva*.

> *Looking for your light,*
> *I went out:*
> >   *it was like the sudden dawn*

of a million million suns,
a ganglion of lightnings
for my wonder.
O Lord of Caves,
if you are light,
there can be no metaphor.[3]

In yoga, full liberation or eternal beatitude is known as *kaivalya*: being separated from all illusions and resting in the natural state. It dawns in sahasrara when the seed-uniting consciousness of ajna is sustained in samadhi (when attention is fully absorbed within the Source realm of consciousness). In the full liberation of kaivalya, the erotic mysteries of death and after death open, as immortality takes on an awesome, crystalline reality.

TRANSFORMING PASSION INTO DIVINE RAPTURE

Thus the yogic ars erotic details of anatomy reveal otherwise mysterious and often underappreciated dimensions of both physiological and spiritual transformations. An observation made from the more scientia-slanted perspective of *ayurveda*, yogic medical physiology, provides a somatic-ecological basis of respect for the seed forces of human procreativity and bodily harmonies:

The food we eat is transformed into the seven body constituents (dhatus) by an involved step-by-step transformation process. The digested food is successively converted into lymph, blood, tissue, fat, bone, marrow, sexual secretions, and an eighth constituent called ojas—subtle light energy. The ojas, the most refined essence of the sexual secretions, in turn permeates and nourishes every cell of the body. With an increase in ojas there is a marked increase in well-being at all levels. With a loss of ojas everything deteriorates. The development of each bodily constituent is directly influenced by the one preceding it. Therefore, if an excessive amount of sexual energy is lost (loss of sexual energy happens mainly through sexual activity) the production of ojas suffers. . . . There is an excess of sexual secretions produced each month to allow for one monthly intercourse without detriment to physical, mental, emotional and spiritual well-being.[4]

Seen in this light, urdhvaretic brahmacharya reflects the inexorable yogic rhythms of our anabolic biochemistry and fertility cycles (for both men and women, though some sources are not specific regarding female orgasmic rhythms, based in the obvious retas differences between the genders). While the quota of one orgasm per month can appear repressive when compared with the statistical averages in the United States, where sex or masturbation is often a daily practice, the personal question is whether we might be overconsuming our own potent seed energies, which underlie maturations into entheogenic ojas, amrita, virya, auras, and nirbija-samadhi.

In the upward glow of urdhvaretas, the radiant beauty of ojas being matured in manipura can reawaken Mother Kundalini from where she "went to sleep" in muladhara after completing her motherly gestation of the zygote, embryo, and fetus to the stage of viability, long ago in our mother's womb.* Upon her awakening, the deepest of charismatic maturational processes begin to unfold as she further matures all bodily energies or pranas in what is called pranotthana (uplifted life energy). This can be accompanied by movement in the form of shaking, quivering, trance-dancing, davening, zikr-rocking, and as sahaja (spontaneous) asanas and mudras unfolding endlessly, for hours, thus evoking openings or puberties in each of the chakras. As entheogenic pineal orgasmic capacities emerge within this whole-bodied charismatic awakening, previous concerns or attachment to frequencies of genital orgasm relax even further.†

Khechari mudra, literally, "lingual delight gesture in the spaciousness of ultimate openness" is one of the most matured ars erotica puberties. In this most mysterious unfoldment, the tongue weaves back into

---

*To enter deeper into this mystery, see the meditation "Retas Mysteries" in chapter 7.
†To see examples of spontaneous mudras and asanas, see 4:35–5:15 and 7:29–8:35 www.youtube.com/watch?v=VlY-DecXk-o.

the throat in response to, and in warm hopes of, making contact with the moonlike allure of the pineal gland (which corresponds to ajna chakra, the site of the third eye). Passion reaching up from the entrails arouses the tongue in a range of tumescences, in dialogue with the now arousable midbrain glands. Glossolalia and all worldwide forms of spontaneous sacred chanting are its precursors and midwife.

Through a serene suspension of breathing, heat is generated within the frenulum and mindspace to the point of an "alchemical" awakening in various glands and chakras. After many years of development, khechari mudra will culminate in the secretion of amrita, or "immortality nectar," a composite of rejuvenating, natural entheogenic-psychedelic essences, the emotion-"moon" juices, and radiances of consciousness. Herein lies the significance of Shiva's crescent moon and the jutting of a cascading river out of the top of his head as seen in many of his images.

Mother Kundalini's adult, postbirth, continuation of the gestational process via all these meditative, charismatic, and ecstatic phenomena is not a regressive "return to the womb." It is a retas-infused extension of the dramatic intensity of that nine-month time of body-manifestation toward extraordinary levels of maturation. For some few, ten or more hours per day of charismatic processes unfold for decades, should outer support exist for such a rare yogi who then blesses the world with shaktipat from her closeness to the Source energies. Over the course of many incarnations, the confluence of matured rasas, khechari, *vajroli* (upward, xylemic blossoming tumescence of the urethra), *shambhavi* (tumescent delight gesture of eyes and sight), and *unmani* (cerebral tumescence of mindspace) mudras, and completed retas activations of nirbija-samadhi, the saint-yogi births herself into the *divya sharira,* divine light body. (See the "Saint" section of chapter 13 for more on this extremely rare stage of urdhvaretic maturity.)

Using the criteria given in Jnaneshvar's commentary on the *Bhagavad Gita,* it has been approximately seven hundred years since any Indian yogi has experienced this complete bodily maturation and transformation:

XIV. Serene and fearless, firm in the [pathways of urdhvaretas brahmacharya] subdued in mind, let him sit, harmonized, his mind turned to Me and intent on Me alone. . .

259. So appears the body (of the yogi) when Kundalini has drunk of the nectar, and even the god of death is afraid to look at it.

260. Old age vanishes, the knot of youth is loosened, and the lost bloom of childhood reappears.

261. Whatever his age, the word "youth" should be interpreted as "strength," such is his incomparable fortitude.

262. Just as the ever new jewel-buds open on the boughs of a tree of gold, fine new finger-nails grow;

263. new teeth appear, very small, set like rows of diamonds on each side.

264. Over the whole body tiny new hairs spring forth like small splinters of rubies.

265. The palms of the hands and feet are red as lotus flowers and in the eyes there shines an indescribable lustre.

266. As the shell of an oyster no longer holds the pearl when it is fully developed and it bursts open at the joint with the force of its growth,

267. so the sight, which strives to pass outwards when it cannot be held within the eyelids, embraces the whole heavens, even with half-opened eyes. . . .

272. She [Kundalini] is the Mother of the worlds, the glory of the empire of the soul, who gives shelter to tender sprouts of the seed of the universe,

273. the phallic symbol of the formless Brahma, the containing vessel of Shiva, the supreme soul, and the true source of the life breath. . . .

291. 'One body devours another.' This is the secret of the teaching of Natha, but it has now been revealed by Sri Vishnu.[5]

These are some, but not all, of the most secret teachings of yoga. Some rest partially hidden in the metaphors in the above sutras. Others are surrounded by a protective "twilight" secrecy inherent to ars erotica pedagogy (see chapter 12 on "twilight" teachings); certain teachings, we are told, cannot be revealed except when the aspirant is fully ready and in need of them. Sir John Woodroffe, an early translator of yogic texts, recounts:

> Copies of the complete tantra are rare enough. . . . I came across a complete manuscript some two years ago in the possession of a Nepalese Pandit. He would, however, only permit me to make a copy of his manuscript on the condition that the Shatkarma Mantras were not published. . . . I was unable to persuade him [otherwise].[6]

Such protection is not unwarranted, as evidenced in the widespread dilution of yogic terms such as kundalini, advaita, guru, or samadhi in popular Western usage. In this singular way, an intimacy surrounds certain erotic truths with living trust. Others are quite simply ineffable.

MEDITATIVE KNOWING

Dharmaviruddho bhutesu kamo 'smi . . .
I am the passion in beings aligned with universal harmonies
(that unfolds complete maturation and enlightenment)

BHAGAVAD GITA

Fortunately, not all the secrets of yogic ars erotica are hidden from view. Meditation has, for thousands of years and millions of people, formed a pathway to freedom marked by an influx of joy and creativity; it has the power of awakening the perineal-to-pineal puberties that form the bodily basis for ars erotica lovemaking, inner marriage, and more. Through eros-enthralled meditation we are able to transcend our more problematic preoccupations with success or failure or pain and pleasure, far beyond all cynical or demystified certainties.

When meditation is retas-infused, the wisdom of worldly procreational and relational life floods in. A world of inner-light radiances, dispassionate beauties, and trans-physical realities emerges, along with myriad bodily tumescences called sahaja asanas, mudras, and anahata-nad utterances. You see the retas-connected enlightenment that was shining brightly from the lives of the tens of millions of yogis who've come before us, recorded in numerous yogic and Buddhist texts. Your meditative awareness is no mere "being present in the Now," unwittingly saturated in scientia myopia. Your awareness is rasa-saturated with the ars erotica wisdom of the ages and you esteem mother, father, seed, spinal puberties, and new-to-dying life of everyone with utter reverence and empathic understanding.

Meditation: The Silent Partner to Conventional Sex

Even sexologists note that a primary reason conventional sex feels so good is that we become expectation-free "sensual meditators" during that time, and it is the receptive focusing of our attention upon the stimulations of sex that makes the pleasure available to us. Who can tell what the innovative sexologist John Money is referring to in the following description?

> The two minds drift into the oblivion of attending only to their own feeling, so perfectly synchronized that the ecstasy of the one is preordained to be the reciprocal ecstasy of the other. Two minds, mindlessly lost in one another.[7]

Although he refers to sexual intercourse, he could just as well be describing what urdhvaretas and meditation expert Swami Kripalvananda has called "the embrace of love-drenched minds" of brahmacharya lovers, heart-to-heart merely looking at one another, or simultaneously thinking of one another while a thousand miles apart. Indeed, William Broad's masturbatory "thinking off" noted in chapter 1 glimmers a scientia sexualis innuendo of this heart-mind-based ars eroticism.

In clinical sexology, desire-filled thoughts that aim too strenuously into the future, better known as "performance anxieties," can sabotage even the most passionate encounter. Sexual dysfunction is often merely a result of the anxiety one can feel if distracted by the *expectation* of impending failure. One is preoccupied with the approaching orgasm, and suddenly and "as usual" it happens too soon. Or one expects the orgasm or requisite arousal *not* to happen, and those bracings for failure impede tumescence and release.

The clinical remedy? "Sensate-focused attention"; that is, a little nonattached, meditative regard for subtlety. Partners touch more slowly, breathe and move with greater relaxation, and even drop the agenda of sex and orgasm-seeking. Unwittingly, sex therapy has moved them infinitesimally toward urdhvaretas!

Meditation Follows the Mystery

The steps across the yogic bridge from sensate focusing's more conventional erotic truths to the subtler ars erotica truths of what we call *consciousness* itself were first put into an ordered format by the great meditator and semanticist Patanjali (200 BCE). In his *Yoga Sutras* (yoga aphorisms), he noted six ever-deepening degrees of sensate focusing: *pratyahara, dharana, dhyana, sabija-samadhi, nirbija-samadhi,* and *kaivalya.*

Pratyahara, "attention that reverses the scattering," gathers us from our wandering opinions, spinning worryings, and jumpy reactions to the myriad external stimulations. The happy or sad story of our relationship or life—constantly replaying itself in our minds with its voice-over analyses, fantasies, and occasional cynical eddies—begins to drop away.

> As an experiment, sit quietly and breathe in and out while making a smooth, hissing sound deep in your throat. Just listen to the sound and let it fill your awareness. Your thoughts will vanish for at least a few moments. This is the beginning of pratyahara.

No longer so tossed about by thoughts, we become capable of a more unbroken perception of each other and ourselves. We pass through the gates of cynical and demystified certainties toward suggestive ambiguity. We hear the songs of inflection beneath speech. We feel the greater whole coming together, previously obscured by our habitual fragmenting preoccupations. Drawing back from the rush, we feel the quieter emotions of shyness, charm, and trepid vulnerability as the graceful but uncertain romanticism of life.

In early pratyahara, even mundane activities approach the sense of being sacred rituals. The poetry of daily life no longer escapes us, the wistful beauties, as one of my most bereft therapy clients once said, "I just want to someday fight traffic with everybody else to get home to my wife and kids . . . someday." For when the mind slows down, we see more rightly with the eyes of the heart. Pratyahara's gaze is also essential to break through the reductive "penis-vagina" mindset of scientia sexualis to be able to see the many retas mysteries in tantric lingam-yoni rituals such as the one described in the "Ritual Worship of Mystery" section of chapter 10.

Pratyahara sustained will intensify, further revealing the finer gradations of evanescent subtleties glimmering within the more dense, suggestive erotic innuendo. This more smoothly alive, impermanent world of self and others appears as if one were experiencing it for the first time, yet repeatedly so. We find one response, feeling, or perspective transmuting into another and another; simultaneously, we know that none of this has ever happened before. The sung mantra reveals myriad shifts in rhythm and sentiment; the in-and-out breath surfaces its manifold textures and inexplicable origin. Thus captivated, our meditation deepens naturally.

Try sitting quietly and practicing the hissing breath, alone or in close synchrony with your partner. Consider: "Each breath is unique, my life is this series of breaths, just like this one, and this one, and . . ."

We may want to linger, to stay, to arrest the flow, and talk about it. Yet this beauty is mercurial and is already slipping away to be replaced by the new. We are getting into the stream-of-living-time.When we step into this temporal flow, our listening gets smooth. We begin to hear sheer hearing itself, the silent sound of one hand clapping; our eyes even close, and we see the light of seeing itself and shambhavi mudra begins to stir; in the movement of breath, we feel bare touching. Something that feels like an underlying profundity is drawing us inward.

We arouse instead into the concentration of dharana, "holding toward unwavering-focus," a nearly continuous nongrasping awareness of the flowing evanescence of mercurial subtleties. The "intelligence" within our intelligence that precedes language breaks through our familiar sense of our "knowing-speaking self." Preoccupying thoughts loosen their grip, and the ensuing silence feels ecstatic. As the fourteenth-century Eastern Orthodox monastic Nicephorus the Solitary advised in a Christian version of dharana:

You know that our breathing is the inhaling and exhaling of air. The organ which serves for this is the lungs which lie round the heart, so that air passing through them thereby envelops the heart. Thus breathing is a natural way to the heart. And so, having collected your mind within you, lead it into the channel of breathing through which air reaches the heart and, together with this inhaled air, force your mind to descend into the heart and to remain there. Accustom it, brother, not to come out of the heart too soon, for at first it feels very lonely in that inner seclusion. But when it gets accustomed to it, it begins on the contrary to dislike its aimless circlings outside . . . so the mind, when it unites with the heart, is filled with unspeakable joy and delight. Then a man sees that the kingdom of heaven is truly within us.[8]

As dharana blooms into full tumescence, one falls devotionally in love with undistracted devotion itself, and the "kingdom within" begins to emerge like a slowly dawning sun. In this unwavering appreciation, a further threshold of wonder opens as dhyana, "fathoming, unwavering attention."

If dharana is a devotional attention like a sometimes smooth, occasionally shifting flow of water, dhyana (meditation proper) is like an unperturbed flow of warm, sacred oils, deep and rich, motionless in its motion. In this depth one begins to feel, as in any portentous first meeting, "*This* is really it! Here it *all* comes together!" We feel the underlying unity of all being, all time, and all people that differentiates into the poignancies and drama of existence.

Thus the Buddha's great enlightenment began one day while he merely watched with heartbreaking compassion the quiet struggles of an oft-pausing, heavy-breathing old man laboring his way down a bustling Indian street. A poignancy so singular and true awakens dhyana to the essence of loving commitment, far beyond the simple dichotomy of pleasure and pain: the constant following of eros-as-mystery unfolding over an entire lifetime in sometimes magnificent, sometimes sorrowful twists and turns.

Subjective attention and all objective manifestation come to a steadiness at their conjoint omphalic source. The solemn sanctity and breathless bliss of this union are exactly that of an engagement for lifelong, no "outs" marriage, known as sabija-samadhi, "complete togetherness with origin-consciousness (samadhi), with seeds (bija) of numerous karmas, powers, and potentials still in the process of activating and expending (sa)." Here, the mind-puberty of unmani mudra also pertains.

After a long-developing engagement of innumerable hours of secret liaisons (thousands of hours a year, for decades), this meditation-marriage of sabija-samadhi consummates in nirbija-samadhi, "complete dissolution into the origin-consciousness, in which the seeds (bija) are completely 'exhausted' (nir)." Fully retas-enriched consciousness, known now as omnidirectional love, or *prema,* opens in a vast embrace.

All the arguing, opposites, demystified certainties, suggestive ambiguities, and evanescent subtleties light up with this singular love song. The scaffoldings (of this book) come down; the entire mystery of consciousness, the retas-infused body, and existence has been revealed.

Finally, after many years or lifetimes of ever-deepening intimacy in this meditative marriage of nirbija-samadhi, the wisely innocent kaivalya, the "natural state," is born. This state of fully liberated erotic life is the utterly new beginning, unencumbered by the laborious and consuming processes that have borne it—sheer trust, a gift, a "virginal-born" spirit, living without reservation in self-world intimacy, where mystery is the deepest, for even the seeming terminus of death has yielded to the endless mystery.

A Moment of Silence . . .

Without awe and pause-taking, we can race past the aura of profundity that looms heavy whenever great erotic mysteries are approached. Instead of humbling us like some rarely seen velvety orchid, these deep yogic teachings blur pejoratively into apparent new-age jargon. As Malebranche said in the seventeenth century while considering the most interior aspects of human fertility, "One [is rightly in awe] that we penetrate too deeply into the smallest works of God."

Through humbled reverence, the half-understandings of arrogance and the demeanings of cynicism wither. Or rather, humbled reverence is the response that denotes we have touched the hems of mystery, while its absence guarantees we are as yet too assuming, and thus too distant, from its powers. "For Beauty's nothing but beginning of Terror we're still just able to bear . . ." as Rilke says in his *Duino Elegies*. If yoga makes you shudder, then you are feeling its true depth.

The tens of millions of individuals, no different from you or me, who have spent whole lifetimes exploring, guided by these practices and beliefs, at first on faith alone, are due our respect. Their parents, children, husbands, wives, and supportive friends and teachers must be remembered and honored as well. The challenges we will face, surely these yogis also faced, and the encouragement they received from others, we most certainly will equally need.

6
Commitment and Marriage as Grihastha Mysteries

There can be no maturity worthy of the supreme term *enlightenment* without deep fathoming of the retas seed forces of life. For most folks, home and lifelong creative family love is the emotional surround in which higher levels of maturation will best blossom, when uplifted to ars erotica heights, the dynamics of which can be glimpsed in the following.

> *I knew that what you said heart-red*
> *meant what you heart-red said*
> *and that you believed what burst from my lips*
> *was truth burst forever more*
> *with us in the center,*
> *life unfolding into its outer-rings*
> *with urdhvaretas seething into us from another center*
> *deeper still*
> *the choosing: you me, me you*
> *interdependent, a bond forever forth,*
> *a surety of each other's joy in each other's*

superlative yes!
at the mere sight feel sigh smell disarray taste
of each other.

Everywhere drip urges to go nowhere else
homing in, the ancient enshrining of the
two-as-one-flesh,
Uroboric, twining together, two serpents regenerating
each other,
feeding on each other's embodied love,
they grow by giving and feeding, this way, that way,
called "devotion," called "marriage," called "home,"
infinitely sustainable.
Another round of believing upon another of knowing,
beautifying, empowering, adoring,
the interplay between them flicking back and forth,
receiving love with gratitude given back that beautifies
both only more.
And he knew her and she him.
Only always compelled deeper into marriage within
marriage within—
but endangered, always,
for, going incrementally further into the merging
oneness,
—our sustained meditation—
all relies upon the other
who relies upon him
relying upon her.
HerHimHerHimHerHim

Some examples from my professional experience also eloquently demonstrate the dimensions of life that can open for us all.

I was leading a pariyanga retreat at Moscow Aquarian Age Yoga Center when a young wife confided to us all that she would bring her husband's shirts to her face to breathe in his fragrance whenever he was away for very long and everyone burst into tears, including the humbled husband.

I was guiding a group of Indian spouses in Chennai in the sharing of admiration when a twenty-year-married wife divulged that for fifteen years she secretly took in extra cleaning tasks to hide away money for their child's education someday, whereupon her husband burst into tears, saying, "I never knew that you were doing this for our [daughter] Priya!" whereupon his wife welled up with tears as she said, "But, yes, it is my duty to do so," whereupon I suggested, "And now you are allowing the divinely human admiration of your husband to nourish you," whereupon she said, "Thank you, Amit, for admiring me as mother and for what I did for our daughter. But, you do the same for our family at your shop, and I would like to tell you that more often." (To me:) "You know, Dr. Sovatsky, in India we don't express such things that are our duty, we just do it and go on."

I was in a thatched-roof, earthen-floor home for seven children, parents, and an elderly lady who was lying motionless on a mat outside. "Is this your Grandma?" I asked one of the kids, "Yes, she is our devotion to Lord, she is dying," he sadly answered.

We need to replace both the scientia sexualis pathologization of the family and the neo-spiritual condescension in which "family life is mere mellow-drama" with "family as divinity become flesh." Hear the words of one woman describing her and her husband's beautiful evolution.

> I worked with Gary for two years before he ever asked me out. He was just one of the guys in our office. Then I found out about his adventures living in Spain, his family, and pet quirks. After we slept together, seeing him in the office was never the same. How could I have even thought of him as the nondescript figure I passed in the hall? After we got married a year later, those images seemed even more bizarre. When Gina was born, I wondered if she had been hiding somewhere between us in the halls or at the watercooler.
>
> Thirty years later, Gina and her husband, Tony, made Gary and me grandparents with the birth of Alexandra, our first grandchild. My parents, in their nineties, had a glow in their eyes between tears of joy

and utter disbelief that their lineage was rippling forth, even as they were largely incapacitated last year when we brought Alexandra to meet them. My Mom even said, "I wish my parents were here to see little Alexandra!" Then Dad chimed in, "I am thinking of my Grandpa Archie, who would be around 160 years old right now; I can see his face lighting up just as if he was here now, just like I remember when he first saw his granddaughter, Beth—Yes, you, Beth!—for the first time!" When Dad said that, looking at me with his eyes wider than saucers, he launched me into an eternity of love and family that I feel just as strongly, now, even though Dad has been gone since last spring. God, almighty! It's like he's in this room right now, taking a peek into her buggy!

Then there's Al and Ronnie—unable to conceive—who decided to volunteer four months each year at an orphanage in Haiti, where they ended up adopting a baby that is now fifteen years old, living in the United States with her mom and dad. They just went back to Haiti to connect her with her roots in a different sort of "brave new world" family.

Here is how it blossoms:

> *You straightened my tie that morning "just," you said,*
> *"to look at me a little longer." Remember?*
> *Your precise fingers shaping the knot,*
> *centering it, looking straight into my eyes,*
> *that moment passed too quickly,*
> *chosen, given over to each other,*
> *it passed in wider circles in other houses,*
> *thatched-roof cabanas, yurts, split-levels,*
> *where there are couples just like us,*
> *enjoying reluctantly preparing to separate each morning . . .*
> *You felt finally like part of the world, you wrote me,*
> *the departures for offices, harvests, hospitals, wars,*
> *factories, trucks, freighters—not wanting to part,*
> *already feeling the missing,*
> *and before that not wanting to get out of bed*

your head on my chest breathing in breathing out,
    perfect—

For what is love but this
uncertain flickering impermanence
embraced as it slips away
re-grasped this way then that,
through persistence, romantic ardor,
surrenders to us hints of the infinite
when we care enough for those whom we love,
against all odds, to worship each and all,
till, pausing, with finger pressed to one's own lips
while preparing to express something of it again,
no next inhalation finally comes?

In contrast, see Mary, who at thirty-eight wants Bill, thirty-one, to "get committed," to choose marriage, children, and a home. Bill says he isn't ready; he wants to travel; he isn't sure. Two years go by. Mary is forty, and Bill is thirty-three: no house, no marriage or children, and no travel. Their "commitment" has been to expectations as ideas and place markers for the future. The *idea* of "family" intimidates Bill and gives Mary a sense of certainty in what she wants, while Bill's "traveling" intimidates Mary and gives Bill a place marker for his future. Then, having become very aware of their "patterns" and interlocking "games," they awaken to the actual power of their shared fertility and begin to feel "invincible" and start getting very creative about how to "make it all work."

The extramarital affair of Carol and Ed reveals a different kind of elusive gamble with mystery and certainty. Carol and Ed are in different marriages. Their affair with each other feels "filled with possibilities" and is a relief from the grind of expectations in their respective marriages. In six months they divorce their spouses and begin living with each other, and in two more months they are pregnant.

We understand their feeling of the magic of possibilities born during their affair, but we wonder whether they will be able to stay committed to possibilities or whether a life of expectations will reemerge.

Will the spiritual ambiguities and paradoxes of finitude and infinitude that were awakened in their affair be shared with awe in their marriage, or will these profundities be trivialized in the anxieties of daily life? Will they join the 60 percent of second marriages and 70 percent of third marriages that end in divorce? Or might they awaken to the ars erotica's powers, with the recognition that their first marriages could just as well have "worked," too, if only they had "known."

Ars erotica commitment is the very nature of human relationships. Commitment, then, is an active meditation on the possible—the retas seed mysteries ever more unfolding their many puberties, enlightenments, new and aging lives—all needing our care, as we are nourished by them, in an interconnected ecology of love. See how it manifests:

Names learnt, work and friends' lives followed,
health conditions, nieces' birthdays, money woes,
who said what—remembering all this is devotion,
is consciousness given and received,
the ultimate, while doing dishes, homework, whether we
    know it or not.
These will be the concerns we have worried too much over
such is life in our patch of the universe.
It vanishes except we listen, care, respond.

The glory of it all at the end,
in the distance ahead, crowning golden—
we will one day vanish, ethereal,
into the murmuring shadows between the slender trees.

Lives weaving into weavings into sangha (community),
the dark night fire burning down in the center of a circle
toward embers of perfect couples,
the children in their own circle playing with long sticks in
    the fire,
the elders, our parents, their grandparents already
    wandering mindless,

drifting heedless, blending into the forests
(someday, us . . .),
blessing us with their rounded backs,
watching us as they trudge up the ancient hillside,
now above us, looking back down,
wincing at the beauty of us all beneath them,
soon to be left behind.

The deeper the perception, the deeper the commitment, which is to say the less it can be ended by any event. The most daring perception—being the resilience, beauty, and creativity of the embodied soul—awakens devotional commitment. Such depth allures us with its loyalty and comforts, as much as its silent foreshadowing of our own mortality awes and frightens us.

The unknown future draws us into keeping our erotic commitments. The retas seed energies of lifelong maturation give us what we need each step of the way. The mystery of it all draws us on suspensefully, the retas possibilities of more proficient communication, more maturity, more growth, more love, and more joy. If we camouflage the sense of the unknown future by premeditating a life of expectations to be achieved, or the cynical certainties of "more of the same old shit," then we can lose touch with the magnetism of this mystery. Fear and suspense are not enemies but allies (albeit precarious ones), which indicate that the erotic mystery of the unknown future is alive to us. All relational planning for the future must make room for such erotic fear and not try to plan it out of existence.

All sorts of difficulties can befall us, but couples living within the intimus will go through them in ever more intimate closeness and sharing. "For better or for worse, till death do us part" is not an obligation; it's an honor. When the spinal puberty activates, it is as if the kundalini goddess of life has rewarded our efforts of loyalty through the thick and thin of daily life, our yogic ars erotica practices in harmony with the rising sun, our constant interpersonal worship and erotic playfulness (known as lila in the emotional bhakti yoga traditions). Then the entheogenic nectars flow down through the mind into our throats, which are choked with tears at the poignancy of life and the wonder of the now-revealed depths of wisdom and ecstasy in human bodies and fully matured erotic relationships.

Each step along the way, from the first moments of attraction to the decision to live together or marry, is guided by a mystery whose possibilities need and allure our attention. When we plant a seed, we do not water it merely because of a stated agreement but because the mysterious potential within its fertility calls us to water it. When the watering is a chore, our union with the seed is *viyogic,* or hidden from us, and when joyful, it is *yogic,* or revealed to us.

In both states we relate to the seed as the mystery of hidden potential that it is and as the mystery of care that we are. Both cynical resentment and enjoyment can lead us to the romanticism of the mystery, if we shift to the intimus. Losing the sense of erotic mystery, however, can easily lead to a withering neglect, usually leaving a trail of last-ditch efforts of guilt-inducing expectations and ultimatums, where divorce becomes a demystified "certainty" that "makes perfect sense." To keep commitment alive we need to perceive the ongoing mystery of things, speak it into words, and activate it as deeds of increasing responsibility.

In erotic mystery we exchange the weight of commitment and the debate of whether or not there is enough of it in a relationship for the more subtle and dynamic task of being loyal to what is mysterious in each other as the source of possibilities. Conclusive, judgmental, past-oriented, or critical thinking that covers erotic mystery with its projective determinations must again and again give way to the hope beneath the dashed hopes, the suspense of our own continuations.

We need to cultivate the support given to us by our partners or spouses so as to quicken all the retas creativities within ourselves to be born as family-community care and right livelihood within this suffering world. No word of encouragement from a partner should remain fallow in us, but should be passionately catalyzed into many creative blossoms of love and work. The world needs more heart-centered highly creative professionals of all sorts, in the one world family, from all the world's Wall Streets to all the Main Street and village paths, everywhere.

So-called fear of commitment is really "awe of the possible," which has been crushed under the weight of a contractual ideal of commitment defined by expectations. Here is the source of nearly all diversions from mystery, such as manipulation, abuse, lying, neglect: mistaking the awe of the possible for the fear of the previously expected.

The mistake throws us backward, and we, tragically, wobble, then run away, looking for explanations (which serve as a kind of ex post facto expectation, as in "I should have *known* it wouldn't work"). Too typically, the relationship becomes primarily an analytic game between two amateur (and now, cynical) psychotherapists. They miss the callings of erotic mystery as their analytic machinery sends them whirring into the past, seeking causal-explanatory certainties for the difficulty. "Awesome mystery of marriage? Oh, sure! With my childhood, it's no wonder; and now *this* difference between us! This whole thing is one big mistake!" was Martin's disparaging statement on the stressful eve of his own wedding. But truly, hasn't each move, from the first date to tuxedo rentals, been an awesome mystery followed forward?

Awe or fear, a nuance within a nuance. But the difference made in choosing between these two word-cousins to describe erotic matters could be all the difference in the world. We hear such a quiet tone-setting in the nuances that distinguish "possibility" from "expectation"; that is, between the allure of an awesome mystery and the eager hopefulness of a well-defined demand.

For example, Ann and Mike improve their communication skills through therapy and by reading several books. They both find it much easier to clearly express their expectations of each other. When they begin to understand the spiritual context of erotic mystery, their recently improved skills reveal the deeper meaning of their efforts as expressions of the magical feeling of "all is possible for us" that they felt when they first fell in love. These feelings nourish their relationship and are what they really want to communicate about and share. This magical mood makes them feel "more alive" and aware that their time "here" is limited. But even the sense of a limited lifetime only serves to add a hallowing tint to their sharings. How so? Retas is the very reservoir of "future aliveness."

The side effect of a prolonged commitment to a relationship as an unfolding mystery is doubly awesome. First, we must not be afraid to call such commitment by its towering name: ever-more unconditional love. Second, we must be able to say that we have learned to need and be needed by a particular and noninterchangeable other, recognizing that sustained need individualizes us with its maturing, unifying, and deepening passion.

LIFELONG COMMITMENT: THE CRUX OF FINITUDE

The anxious image of a ticking reproductive clock, fearful signs of midlife crises, concerns about money for now and later, and regressively hopeful preoccupations with the metaphor of the "lost inner child" are all modern, troubled reactions to the forward movement of life. In a demystified world, a materialistic interpretation often prevails, and nothing profound informs life's difficulties with layers of wonder. In family life the finite resources of tasks per day, dollars per year, and topics per discussion begin aligning with one economic interpretation of the erotic mystery or another. Fights about money, about getting the toy everybody else has, or about what was or wasn't said, which flare up so often in family life—what surrounds such passions? The poignancies of an impermanent mystery fading into the edges of the infinite.

Time, money, and speech should be demigods of sorts; that is, permeated with a challenge to feel their awe. A counseling client looks in his wallet to pay me. His hushing silence and trepid movements are as though he is entering a chapel. His payment to me is a painful, sacrificial offering, and, suddenly faith-shaken, he is unclear about what he is receiving from me in return. Beneath perfunctory nods of "thank you," "you're welcome," a mystery of doubt, faith, hope, and survival passes, then some calmness surfaces.

Marriage, monogamy, and lifelong commitment are not goals or securities but rather the natural results of two partners sensing the depths of the possibilities within each other. We find that we need the time of a lifetime to fulfill all that is suggested by what we see and how we feel. Fear of and attraction to lifelong monogamy (or even lifelong loyal polyamory) are reflections of the awe of the possibilities between any two people who see each other so deeply, for in feeling the need for the time of the rest of our lives, the finitude of it all quickens. Such is the fructifying nature of need. Can the north and south poles of a magnet leave each other? This is our gender profundity! And it includes the inner marriage, from perineum to pineal, as well.

Deep rhythms vibrate through us whenever we grasp the truths of life and align with them. The sense of a finite, aging lifetime is one such truth, an embodied, erotic truth. Perhaps as we die, at whatever age, we receive a last awakening, remarking to ourselves, "So *that* was what a lifetime is all about!" As the organic wholeness or grace of the finite, singular lifetime is grasped one way and then another over the years and decades of our lives, it provides a fundamental sense of the range of human possibilities and can stimulate our involvement. Such is the way of maturation.

The twenty-year project of raising a family (or the forty-year project of a grand-family) is another organic time span. As one Chinese proverb has it, marriage is complete on the birth of the first grandchild. As ars erotica fully blooms its puberties of heart-mind, you can see that divorce, serial monogamy, cyberporn, and broken families (or those who merely rail against such things, as well as against abortion, gay marriage, and so on) are for people living in the scientia sexualis that is almost everywhere else. You and yours are living "in a different economy of bodies and pleasures," as Foucault smiles upon us from the *antara-bhavas,* in poignant delight.

Then, "staying married for the sake of the children (and grandchildren)" suddenly loses its drudgery and cynical cast. Instead, for you and your ars erotica friends, the wholeness of three or four generations of life, all together, uplifts you within the glowing intimus: "Of course, get help, stay together for the kids and the grandkids, and maybe great-grandkids, too—that's where the gold is!"

A wistful poignancy infuses the days for Margaret, ninety-four, and Bill, ninety-six, with the slow and undeniable approach of maha-samadhi, the great return to the Source, looming ahead. In their Gentle Yoga class, they learned that they are in the range of the one-hundred-year ideal yogic life, along with their nearly unbroken lineage of five children (four in lifelong marriages, and one still struggling), eight grandchildren (seven in their original marriages, too, and one in her second marriage), and then there are the great-grandchildren.

Then, hospice is called in for Margaret. Bill, her husband of seventy-four years, is there and their five adult children, all now themselves gray-haired elders in their seventies and sixties (whose naked, crying births Margaret easily recalls when she and Bill were "just starting out," over seventy years ago!). All eight of her "adorable little grandchildren," now in their fifties and forties (some of whose births she also distinctly recalls, as if just yesterday!), and their spouses are there, too. And yes, the four great-grandchildren are there, from early twenties to eighteen, all of whom are "just starting out." Indeed, then there is little wriggling and gazing-about Mattie, the youngest great-grand-kid, and pregnant Rochelle, sitting nearest to her bed.

Margaret's grihastha enlightenment is incomparable; it ripples through her family around her—the continuity of life that more than "seems" to stretch on and on into the future—nothing could be more indelible for her than the prospect that her soon to be left behind family tree will go on and on, after she is, well, "not here." Indeed, she recalls her own parents and grandparents and their faded-away stories of their parents and grandparents, all long gone. "You are the heart of my life," Margaret says as she smiles and cries, "May you all go on forever!"

Can there be any doubt that the profundity of the grihastha enlightenment, comprised of day-to-day struggles, gratitudes, crises, forgiven breakdowns, and ever-deepening loyalties—is "well worth it, every day," and, climactically, on some wistful "final day," way into the future?

TO STAY OR TO LEAVE?

Before breaking up, people often say they are "dying" in their relationships. Confusingly, in such situations one is hard pressed to determine how much of this feeling of dying is being induced by one's considered withdrawal from the relationship, by some deficiency in the relationship, or merely by an unavoidable inkling of one's own mortal nature.

"Should I get out or should I stay?" Once raised, the question seeks an answer, while also pervading the relationship with precariousness and impossibility, even from the earliest moments: "He was late, *obviously* irresponsible!" "She was impatient, I don't need *that!*" Some partners fall into a chronic mode of seeing the other as if through the lens of a high-powered psychological microscope and then wonder why their beloveds look so ill at ease. Of course, it takes some time for them to see themselves as peering at their partners in this hypercritical way and to wonder if such peering induced any of the immaturity or insecurity that they identified.

Like many soldiers, each can adapt to these battle-alert conditions and find a certain cynical enjoyment in how well they see each other's faults and how good it feels to point them out and have them pointed out. It feels so good because now the sweetness of righteous anger or even passive-aggression can be wielded by these partners, each waiting in ambush for the other to commit an error that can be pointed out, that supports their developing theory, and so on, mounting expectantly to the dark orgasm of an enraged breakup. This is the shadowy side of the erotic mystery of shared gender, the sharing of the desperate powers of destruction and threatened survival.

Through serial relationships and all that we may have learned from friends, experts, or our parents' martial-marital skillfulness (and they from their friends, and so on), we begin to accumulate our own questionable skillfulness in chronically, perpetually, raising this question of "staying or going," and in assessing the "workability" of a relationship. All such accumulated skills, especially when silently wielded, gnaw away at the possibilities within each other.

Only renewed innocence and awakening to our retas seed potentials can approach mystery and fully imbibe its nourishing allure. But innocence is infinitely renewable, and thus we are rightfully afraid of its power to make things work out, no matter how dysfunctional and horrific a situation. We are returning to that which we, in our critical moments, were so sure was a kind of endless hell, and no doubt we are still deathly afraid of a resolution that would be "too good to be true." If we believed in such a possibility, we would only go back to our partner again, innocently hoping for the best—a foolish move, says our more clever and "experienced" voice. We become caught in a paradox created by too much "knowledge" and not enough retas, energy, maturity, and refreshing innocence. The guidance of an experienced ars erotica mentor can help maximize forward movement at such critical junctures.

As a defensive maneuver, we might find ways to diminish our partner's unique value to us (or to diminish our imagined unique value to him, in order to minimize any potential loss in the future—often before the relationship has even "begun"). Ironically, this might occur just as his value begins to touch the highest levels we've ever allowed ourselves to feel for anyone. We cannot imagine valuing anyone *that* much, or that "it" (that feeling of total possibility) could ever last for very long. We can even mistake evanescent subtlety for cynical "proof" that it won't last. "It" never does. But with retas energies alive, we "keep coming up with the goods" with one another and for one another. "Go for it," retas says, over and over. "Break your bond with alcohol, with procrastinations, with 'associations' from the 'psychoanalytic past.'"

We may hover before the burning bush of each other's mercurial, inestimable mystery, taking in as much of this radiance as our faith (or our various fears of "dependency") permits. We dare to value each other just enough to stay but not so much as to be overly threatened by the specter of his or our leaving. One heartens, the other looks away; the other reconsiders, the one has just given up. Thus, the depths of erotic sharing recede from us, for how can we worship what we will not allow to move us to the point of irreversible devotion and continued, lifelong, retas awakenings?

Innocence is far more powerful than the knowledge born of our fear of past difficulties repeating themselves into the future. Innocence is more creative than any well-reasoned justifications or ideas on how to make things work. It is what gives inspiration to such ideas in the first place. Thus, in the realms of erotic mystery, the question "Should I go or stay?" transforms into a koan and, like the well-known enigma of "the sound of one hand clapping," has no literal answer.

As we wonder "How could this be?" with ever-deepening innocence, our feelings of blame, anger, endangered hope, and hurt become more sharable and less a matter of accusations and rebuttals. When we feel a sense of wonder slip into our worries and problems, we lighten up, we "enlighten." The retas energy we were spending worrying about the "right" choice is returned to our awareness as a feeling of creativity and empowerment. We see possibilities where we once thought there were none. This is not a mind trick; it is the mystery of urdhvaretas, kundalini profundities, and the many powers of consciousness, far beyond simply "being in the Now."*

VIYOGA (HIDDEN UNIONS) AND SPOKEN PASSION

*Better than meeting
and mating all the time
is the pleasure of mating once
after being far apart.*

*When he's away
I cannot wait
to get a glimpse of him.*

---

*For more on enlightened creative knowing powers, far beyond the mere "inner stillness" overly focused upon in the West, see enlightened *avandhana* "learning-mind" saint Dr. R. Ganesh (http://en.wikipedia.org/wiki/Dr._R._Ganesh). Yet what most impressed me about Dr. Ganesh was his choice to care for his suddenly ill mother instead of giving his scheduled, limelight keynote at the World Family Conference in Delhi.

Friend, when will I have it
both ways,
be with Him
yet not with Him,
my lord white as jasmine?

MAHADEVIYAKKA, IN RAMANUJAN,

SPEAKING OF SIVA

Viyoga refers to that class of erotic unions that are veiled by the more obvious experience of apparent separation. It includes the feelings of missing each other and longing to meet each other. It also includes the angers, frustrations, shames, guilts, hurts, fears, and "problems" that obscure the felt sense of union. Through the unreasonable faithfulness interior to viyoga, all such feelings disguise a hidden union and, within mystery, an ars erotic one.

The feeling of missing each other is usually thought of as merely the pain of separation, while it is actually the felt sense of being in hidden union with someone distant from us. It is the felt cord of emotional connection that transcends spatial proximity and empirical proofs. There is no need to resent missing each other, as any romantic can attest.

Yet most of us must learn and perfect the romantic art of "missing" as a throbbing anticipation and not tighten its difficulty into blame and resentment. In viyoga, calls made to another while apart *express* missing, rather than aiming to end it. As that expert on such matters, Saint-Exupéry's fox, explained:

"It would have been better to come back at the same hour," said the fox. "If, for example, you come at four o'clock in the afternoon, then at three o'clock I shall begin to be happy. I shall feel happier and happier as the hour advances. At four o'clock, I shall already be worrying and jumping about. I shall show you how happy I am!"[1]

Viyoga becomes a velvety array of erotic feelings and communications to be shared, perhaps invisibly, with each other. Synchronous experiences—phone calls, shared nocturnal dreams, and other psychic phenomena—rest within this occult dimension of relationship. Viyoga denotes an unconditional relatedness, reaching beyond time, space, and perhaps even the veils of death.

Missing one another or missing your closeness can also take place when you are in each other's presence but feeling estranged. The challenges of sharing differences can lead to actually believing the demystified claim that "Men are from Mars and women are from Venus." The paradox of feeling close to another *via* obvious "differences" is "viyayoga" (*viyoga,* in transliterated Sanskrit) and it can take place for folks living on any two or more planets. The short route back is to share missing directly, which, seen in each other's eyes, transmutes to a wavering longing and reuniting, for the truth of sharing is already occurring. After "I miss you!" the apologies, forgivenesses, logistics, and details of the problem can then be worked out together.

Getting into each other's shoes without flitting back to one's own point of view can give rise to a beautiful moment in which you each "get" the other's viewpoint so deeply that you experience uncertainty and even confusion. Your partner's view feels so credible to you that you begin to think she might be right! And your partner gets into your shoes just as deeply and you see it on her face. You know you were "heard." What a gift to see your partner totally inhabit your idea or point of view or choice. What a gift of "feeling competent at empathy" it is to see your empathy "work," as your partner thanks you profusely for getting into her shoes. But retas potentials must still be activated to create solutions and to try them out and refine them, from that point on.

A sense of understanding occurs, perhaps apology and forgiveness and reconciliation, but even then there are hidden levels of deeper relating, such as the inspiring sense of sharing "the exact-same missing" of the one relationship that you are both in, or the spiritual sense of the One Relationship we are all in, or of the shared-gender mystery. Knowing about these more subtle levels of relationship is important, so that we can start missing them and thus spread the depths of human longing to the whole range of our being. These levels, known first as "impossible ideals" or memories of the best of times, become innuendos in the present.

Then, from the detected nuance of some gesture or quivering inflection, an obviously heartfelt reunion floods in: "He got so shy, and I saw who he really is; my forgiveness just came." "Her voice got so soft; suddenly I knew that I had been missing her greatly." Without access to moments of devotional attention directed toward each other, how can these turning points occur? As the reunion occurs, a paradox emerges: all that was "negative" becomes positive proof of the tensile strength of the partners' sharing. What they have just weathered is now becoming an inspirational memory and not a despondent one, as was almost the case.

When we struggle to grasp the erotic magnitude of each single confession, each act of forgiveness, each act of giving or receiving, and each moment of hurt, shame, or anger, then, like Larry, Jill, and Ruth, we can discover the intimacy within viyoga. Larry was making a birthday party for Jill, the twelve-year-old daughter of his girlfriend, Ruth. Larry promised that Jill could invite any eight people to the party. But then a fight occurred between Jill and her mom, and Jill told Larry she didn't want her mom at the party, "and you said I could invite *my* choice." Then Ruth was mad at Larry for letting himself be "manipulated" by Jill and because she was not invited. Larry agreed and felt caught in the middle.

They had spent some hours yelling about their repetitious patterns when Jill apologized to Larry for having manipulated him so as to get back at her mom. Ruth apologized for trying to build a "case" against Larry. Larry agreed with Jill that he should have confronted her with being manipulative and not let her get away with it. They all felt closer, having shared their shame, anger, accusations, apologies, and forgiveness.

Unexpressed gratitude, admiration, and respect are other submerged viyogic unions repeatedly deferred by the habitual conversations of daily life. Sometimes partners will spare their mates their difficulty in receiving compliments by withholding them. Or the recipient shrugs off a compliment with "Oh, it was nothing." Paradoxically, hidden within these perfunctory shrugs are shy waves of gratitude for being acknowledged.

As these communications occur, they provoke unpredictably passionate responses, for shy gratitudes and blushing admirations are the greatest of rasa aphrodisiacs. Such are the glimmers of the soul and the momentarily deeper penetration of the body by their radiant vitality. Often, all that is needed is to begin a sentence with the words "I really admired you when . . ." which is responded to by the simple words "Thank you." Or more fully, "The glowing blush you now see on my face is from receiving your gratitude. This is how much your admiration means to me." Then the other, too, begins to brim up, look, then look away. Too often it seems easier to feel miffed at something lacking than to walk on these quivering viyogic waters toward each other.

Listening to each other (and ourselves) with viyogic artfulness, we will be able to trace envy and jealousy back to admiration and worship; sadness and pity back to compassion; fear, doubt, and suspicion back to the awe of great powers within us and others. Longing, yearning, loneliness, desiring, and missing reveal the viyogic unions during separation, while anger, resentment, grief, disappointment, and hate reflect the anguish of ruptured hopefulness. We can then see shame as a tough-love, usually counterproductive, prod to "shame someone" into becoming a better person, while embarrassment and shyness can be understood as sudden awakenings to one's own visibility and an even greater sense of one's existence.

THE EROTIC FREEDOM
OF BELONGING

In our psychologically sophisticated culture, we are witnessing an over-differentiation and demystification of erotic phenomena that has become xenophobia: the significance of erotic differences made so great as to induce a fearful, confusing, or even hostile sense of foreignness. Looking deeper, we can see that we are drawn together, whether fearfully or alluringly, by something deeper than our differentiating certainties—the mystery of eros. It gathers together all forms of "otherness": genders, erotic preference groups, ethnicities, sexo-political factions. Our humility in the face of the mystery suggests that which is deeper than the freedom of unbridled choices—the seemingly more restricted, but actually more liberating, ecological freedom of belonging to something vast.

In many ways, the freedom of belonging is the highest and most difficult social or world-embracing enjoyment of the erotic mystery. Love becomes the one-embodied-flesh; it is the all-forgiving, long-enduring, and at times excruciating perception of the world as one huge family, where everyone and everything belongs, for no other reason than the fact that we are all here in the same mystery, facing the same unknown.

7
The Passions and Mysteries of Fertility

Unseen buds, infinite, hidden well,
Under the snow and ice, under the darkness, in every
square or cubic inch.
Germinal, exquisite, in delicate lace, microscopic, unborn,
Like babes in wombs, latent, folded, compact, sleeping;
Billions of billions, and trillions of trillions of them
waiting,
(On earth and in the sea—the universe—the stars there
are in the heavens,)
Urging slowly, surely forward, forming endless,
And waiting ever more, forever more behind.

WALT WHITMAN, "UNSEEN BUDS"

The passions of fertility awaken during genital puberty and continue afterward in the approximately monthly cycles of ovulation and spermatogenesis. Throughout most of the rest of nature, the rhythms of these passions orchestrate all sexual behaviors, with many species following cycles or subcycles of the seasons and others in intricate rapport with their own community's fluctuating population densities.

In human societies, fertility and viability have been subjected to all manner of interventions and intentions, ranging from colonization and international wars to tribal fertility rituals, infanticides, and abortions, from arranged marriages and mail-order marriages to shotgun weddings and "love marriages," from planned parenthood with responsible contraception to arduous efforts to conceive via surrogates, sperm banks, and artificial insemination. These intentions have shaped procreative mystery into a "lineage responsibility," an "overpopulation problem," a "biogenetic phenomenon," a "rite of passage into adulthood," a "gender-political problem," an "unintended side effect" or an "intended choice," or the "divine purpose of sex and marriage."

Well-intended shapings of procreativity would perhaps reach their modern technological zenith were a prediction made some years ago by Masters and Johnson to be realized: that even surrogate mothers could be "circumvented entirely by the development of an artificial uterus that maintains the developing embryo-fetus in an incubator-like environment, hooked up to an artificial placenta that functions not unlike a kidney dialysis machine."[1] Such a possibility was grimly envisaged in Aldous Huxley's 1932 classic, *Brave New World,* offering a dark premonition of the insidious losses of human intimacy in a scientia sexualis future. In such a context the sense of a procreative mystery might be felt only by its absence or as translated bizarrely into the "marvel" of cloning or other reproductive technology. In ars erotica future societies, however, hospital maternity wards that today have become more homey "birthing centers" may very well have progressed even further to become temples of sacred birth, adorned for each couple with decors and icons of their own spiritual choosing.

PROCREATIVE WONDERS

What is the actual mystery of our incarnate beginning before any religio-political or scientific theorizings or findings or personal decidings? Along with any literal answers to our question, we hope to recover the actual sense of wonder and awe involved in this mystery. For what seethes within our bodies, although we rarely experience it as such, is the coiled beginning of all future human possibilities. And at some point deep within fertility, all forms of conceptive hopefulness dissolve into a humbling yet exhilarating awe of our situation.

MEDITATION
Retas Mysteries

Repeated empathic reading of these pages will provide you with a supremely profound spiritual meditation, one that can lead into seeds-within-seeds-within-seeds-within-seeds-within-seeds, ad infinitum, back and potentially forward, with all the love and awe this urdhvaretas process deserves. This meditation traces back toward the Source of all life—a "retas dimension" that has manifested every single ensouled body that has ever awakened the cosmic power of the inner male-female union at the base of the spine known as Mother Kundalini. It translates the scientia story of incarnation into that of the yogic ars erotica.

Our journey begins at the oft-defined "beginning": the moment of the sperm-ovum union. But it could just as well begin with the archetypal moment when you were "just a glimmer of attraction" between the man and woman who would become your parents, or when each of them were glimmers of attraction in the eyes of your four grandparents, or they were glimmers of attraction in your eight great-grandparents, and so on.

Meditate slowly and carefully on this:

> Macrocosmic *Ha* (solar-golden) and *Tha* (lunar-silvery)
> life-enhancing outer radiations
> combine with
> microcosmic, inner sun-moon uniting
> ha-tha yoga pre-dawn spiritual practices
> to bless from without and from within
> the embodied maturation of male *shukra* and female *rajas*
> (sperm and ovum forms of retas)
> while their combination in erotic-love-embracing-fertility

catalyzes the womb manifestation of all human life there
     ever was or will be
of course, including
YOU

While scientia sexualis calls your just-conceived body a nonsouled zygote (Greek, *zhog*, "joined together," from Sanskrit, *yoga,* "joined or yoked together"), the *yogaverse* describes you as a soul (the gender-adaptable *jiva*) being drawn from the *antara-bhava* (prebirth dimension) into a particular womb (*yoni*): "the dark, fertile mother-space from whence all consciousness and matter vibrates into earthly existence." Thus, too, the inner darkness of ears-and-eyes-closed meditation is called *yoni mudra.*

You make a three-month-long approach from deepest, fecund soul space to the zygote-maturing-into-embryo. But the heart-awakening rapport is there, long before that. Mother and father may even muse over names for you as boy or as girl during this mysterious and uncertain time.

Within the maturing zygote, the developmental energy within cosmic fecundity called Mother Kundalini provides the energizing, charismatic, "spiritual music" that quivers into the chromosomal, double-helixed strand-dance of meiosis and endless cell-dividing mitosis after the sperm-and-egg union. Thus each of us "is danced" into bodily existence by activated father-mother, sun-moon love.*

This vibratory Mother-music (techno-scientifically called "DNA-information transfer," as if we are all run by computer software) poignantly moves our first divine marriage yoga union (the zygote yogi) into a ball (blastula) that folds into an inner-outer-layered proto-body (gastrula).†

Then, via Mother's deepest kundalini-inspired yoga flow-asanas of all times, the bodily cells get moved, or move themselves, into forming a spine, gut sac, head, brain, mouth, beating heart, arm and leg

---

*http://www.youtube.com/watch?v=aDAw2Zg4lgE
†For a more detailed description, see Sovatsky, "Kundalini and the Complete Maturation of the Ensouled Body."

buds to arms and legs to wriggling fingers and toes in what science calls "embryological gestation." Now those are pretty amazing asanas guided by quite a wise and loving yoga teacher: the father-awakened, Mother Kundalini of all mothers!

Passing through a stage of genital-perineal androgyny, nearly all of us develop into one gender as the other gender's physiology melts into commingled male-female perineal tissues,* adjacent to the root or muladhara chakra where, after quickening your body into existence, Mother Kundalini will dormantly reside in your adult body. But she can be reawakened via sun moon ha-tha yoga to mature you to untold heights.

As your gestation-yoga continues, rudimentary fish gills (pharyngeal arches, reinvigorated in adulthood via yoga's throat-thrusting, *matsyendra-asana* "fish-breathing pose") and a spinal "tail" will also come-and-go, as you retrace billions of years of evolution in what embryological science calls functional or literal "ontogeny phylogeny recapitulation." Amazing!

As your own soul-body connection quickens and deepens, "oxytocin bonding hormones" secrete inside mother's body (and, surely, in correlate secretions in father's body) and your fetal body, creating an embodying, "love-trust connection" between all three of you, months before you are born. The rasa secretion-love-bonding process of oxytocin is the physical-emotional "glue" that holds the entire living universe together.

The completion of bodily quickening coincides with the jiva "glowing itself brighter" from within your very own fetal body. Within all this growth and all this love-intoxicating oxytocin, the Mother and the Father and the jiva get more "up close and personal" with one another and become *your* Mom, *your* Dad and little *you*. For love (or oxytocin, for scientia types) makes people special to one another.

To Mom and Dad, you become "our baby/daughter/son/child" and they become "parents together" with one another. Altogether,

---

*See this amazing Lennart Nilsson photograph of the normal androgynous phase of all human gestations: http://tinyurl.com/mt3w2tn.

the three of you become a family, within an outspreading "family tree" of possible siblings and preceding ancestors, tracing back a million years—yoga would say, tracing back forever.

Thus, your embryogenesis and birth *makes* your parent's parents into "grandparents" and their parents into "great-grandparents" and their parents into great-great-grandparents and so on. Their welled-up tears and quivering moods are the primordial charismatic initiation of each generation into their next wave of matured identity, "I'm a Grandma, I'm a Grandpa!" And everybody else smiles joyfully, deferentially, and is nourished by these so-initiated "elders."

In the ars erotica of yoga and its worship of Divine Mother, Divine Father Prajapati, Lord Prana (life-force), and urdhvaretas seed mysteries, familial love is understood as strong enough to sustain a whole lifetime of connectedness for all concerned for almost all families. Inside of all fetal bodies are the seed potentials for all future seeds— the seed of those seeds—that will become fertilely ripe inside future pubescent bodies. Amazingly, those ripened seeds-within-seeds can combine, decades into the future, with the puberty-ripened seeds of someone who became the other gender—the gender that embryologically melted into androgenous fetal perineal tissues that the two mating male and female persons *still have*! Oh, mystery of gender escapes easy categorization for all!

Then there is the influx of new "genetic material" as each conception blends another lineage into each new, Mother-danced-into-existence, zygote-embryo-fetus-baby. "The world is, indeed, one embracing family," *Vasudhaiva kutumbakam!* sings the ancient Vedic scripture. "Seed-potentials-within-seed-potentials-within . . ." bespeaks the infinity of nested-future-potentials for new lives within you, even before you are born, should other fertile persons erotically love other sperm-egg zygotic yoga-unions into happening with your children, your (and your in-laws') children's children, your children's children's children, and so on.

Within the womb's complex "love-connection chemistry" of entheogenic rasas and umbilical breathing and feeding, you grow through your incarnating, DNA-rasa generated asanas of gestation.

Then you start doing more kicking and poking asanas, indicating that you "want out," around 270 days after your conception via your mother-father's love-bliss union that continues a million years of *Homo sapiens* evolution one more lifetime into the present-future.

From deep within the dark fecundity of the womb, labor contractions joltingly emerge into your mother's body. These charismatic contractions provide your transportation out of the yoni realm via the "birth canal." That is, you are born.

During and thereafter, the oxytocin love-consciousness rasa is conjoined with another entheogenic-juice-essence rasa, known as mother's breast milk; together they keep you nourished, healthy, and happy with Mom after you are born and are "outside," till teeth manifest. At that time, powerful lysomal enzymes lovingly dissolve your gum tissue, as teething (a retas-blossoming rite of passage celebrated by ars erotica parents for thousands of years) occurs, so you can chew earthy foods.*

As a newborn, you continue doing incarnating asanas as you suck and kick and jolt and arch and pull your toes. For a few years you "speak in tongues," enjoying the presemantic pleasures of emotion-development-soundmaking, known as *anahata-nad,* seed-animated, developmental chanting. Everyone else will call it "baby talk" and be charmed, while parents of all times have taken up adult versions of this charming "baby talk" when they call each other "honey," "sweetie," and, of course, "baby." The perfection of how everything fits together could not be made any more romantically perfect, even by the greatest romantic poet of all times!

Concentration on the seed of the seed, ad infinitum, breaks us free of the confines of scientia's self-proclaimed "final liberation," into

---

*By the way, lysomal enzymes will reemerge during your final puberty, known as *khechari mudra,* the yogic gesture of "dancing joyfully from earth-taste realm to heaven-taste realm," around age fifty till death. Then the flesh-dissolving enzymes will lovingly melt away your tongue's frenulum and charismatically bring ars erotic tumescences to your lingual lingam, brain hypothalamus (Greek for "little wedding chamber"), and pineal gland.

the infinitely wider expanse of urdhvaretas. The male-female, totally commingled perineal tissue is the kundalini-triggering point for the heel-to-perineum, cross-legged *siddha-asana* "pose that awakens the cosmic creativities" by causing the totally commingled male-female perineal tissues to have mega-lovers' reunions via thousands of blissful hours of perineal, heart-awakening, heel hugs. This is the core of hatha yoga (not flexibility), as is shown by the oldest known relic of yoga, the Pashupati Seal, which depicts an ithyphallic and ithybreasted yogi in siddha-asana, whose erection has nothing to do with scientia sexualis erections!

Those who go on to awaken their pineal glands into ambrosial puberties get to experience fully matured sex, about five puberties beyond what Freud called "the final maturity of the genital primacy ego!" The profundity of bliss of those who turn ars erotica chakra-keys of perineum, heart, pineal, and mindspace is beyond measure! Mother Kundalini's siddha-asana emerges like birth contractions in its own perfect time to catalyze more of the Mother of the Universe into sending charismatic shivers throughout the yogi's body to cause it to tumesce and twist into all sorts of asanas and thus to feel Mother-Father God in every cell, in every DNA strand, in every molecule in the body.

This is why yoga is fundamentally the path of inner marriages, seed-uniting zygote creation, and endless Shiva-Shakti reunions where fertility-lust-love-body-soul-awe-bliss-maturation-enlightenments are all one "intermingling and maturing" yoga matter.

> *Always oscillating, Shiva worships Shakti worships Shiva*
> *man worships woman worships man*
> *in this escalating circularity,*
> *becoming godlike, becoming goddess*
> *born out of their arduous longing for this other, the beloved,*
> *a weaving maturing of souls verging on oneness,*
> *tangoing flamencoing yinyanging auguring*
> *ever-deeper into the Source of incarnation itself,*
> *close and even closer*

wending weaving winding

toward the vertiginous center

everything quickening the hopes and fears

of each lover there ever was or will be.

CREATING NEW LIFE

The term itself, *procreation,* speaks to the ominous simplicity of conception as a creation—*pro,* on behalf of the divine—not as a biotechnical re-"production" nor as a mere personal intention or social expectation but as a miracle. For procreative choice cannot be reduced to the lone matter of intention to have or not have a child. It is the entrance into the power and wonder of creating life and the uncanny rhythms in which it abides.

Such perceptions are possible only when the specific passions of fertility have been revived, for now fertility is determined largely in deference to the passions of sex desire. Estral cues have all but vanished, while spermatogenesis, or male fertility cycles, remains unexplored; fertility rhythms themselves are, ironically, thought of as either "good" (infertile) or "bad" (fertile) times for sex. Within modern sexual life, fertility has become something we try to "track" when we want to conceive. Even the most well-planned conception or totally controlled artificial insemination does not disguise the fact that we are dealing in mystery and miracle and that participants' intentions circulate at some distance from the realities of conception, gestation, and birth.

Why do people have children? Underneath all the passionate and thoughtful answers, miraculous fertility reminds us that there is no answer. The interrogative should not trick us into seeking the wherefore to this deep why. The matter is a wonder, and conception itself the primal gateway through which all human wondering proceeds. Thus, we will speak less of an intentional conception than of a conscious conception.

During the cyclical peakings of our fertility (the female and the less visible male cycles), we are brought to the very core of the passions of fertility. To share in tantric lovemaking practices of yoga and worship at this time is to sustain the fullness that has been approaching all month in the many subtle nuances of impending ripeness. Perhaps the partners will be especially drawn toward each other and their activation of retas energies will be not only of sexual desire but also of the very energies and images of fertility itself. What is "unsafe time" in the eyes of conventional sex desire appears as awesome possibility in tantric brahmacharya.

Conscious, "miraculous" procreativity and parenthood hover within the relationship particularly during days of fertility and in varying nuances of possibility throughout the fertility cycle, as discovered by Lisa and Rob. After practicing tantric brahmacharya for a few years, they began to experience the passions of fertility as gradual changes in Lisa's complexion and in a subtle "tang" in the odor of their perspirations. Then, during an evening ritual, Rob was receiving Nyasa (described in chapter 10) and began to see a kind of infinite regression of feminine subtleties in Lisa. He felt a slowly turning field of radiance moving around her that made him think of a cornucopia, an endlessly receding vortex that just kept drawing him into her.

Lisa felt her ovaries and womb quivering from time to time, and when she looked into Rob's eyes, her own breath momentarily stopped. She saw an intentness in his eyes, a captivated look that made her feel that "the time" had arrived. As Rob exchanged Nyasa with Lisa, he felt a veil slip away in his contact with her. She rather suddenly became more vivid to him, visually, in her scent, and to his touch. Being practiced in tantric brahmacharya, they allowed their genital arousals to shift through many phases over the following twenty minutes.

During this time, they had a constant, silent experience of embracing each other's thoughts, which were like folds of concern and wonder that kept leading them into quieter depths of each other. Then they heard a buzzing sound, which Rob thought sounded like "the engines of the universe." Together they wondered if this sound was the buzzing of fertility itself that waxed and waned during the lunar cyclings of fertility. While they had previously feared that conceiving and raising a child would be "too difficult" for financial and other practical reasons, now they didn't really know what to do. To follow this experience of their shared fertility seemed worth any expense.

As each month went by, the whole fertility cycle kept inspiring them with its mystery, and all their reasoning and analyses about readiness became inconsequential. They almost broke their brahmacharya on one occasion because the draw toward this fertility was so great, but the bliss and wonder of the sublimation—feeling the godlike power of imminent life procreation—was equally great, and they continued their meditations instead. They decided to approach the procreative mystery together but only in meditative silence.

They then began to feel how little it was up to them yet it was completely up to them. The mystery was dizzying, no longer a thing to merely talk about. There was no decisive way to know beforehand whether or when to leave their brahmacharya. Not until they had shared numerous encounters with the passions of fertility did the following occur: in the middle of a tantric ritual involving the exchange of flowers, they fell into a "pranic mirroring" with each other and began taking off each other's clothes. It felt to them like the "very first time" that not only they but anyone had ever joined genitals.

The sensations were exquisite, no doubt enhanced by the three-year hiatus in genital contact. Every movement was so fresh and alive. They felt each other as "mother of all beings," as "father of all children." Their own fertility seemed to echo inward toward that of their children and their children's children, and on and on. In another way, they felt a proud connection with their parents, grandparents, and a chorus of ancestors who seemed to be smiling delightedly as if some angelic obstetrician had just come into their "waiting room" with the momentous announcement.

They felt on the verge of creation, with everything else in the universe doing this same thing, silently, invisibly, all matter and all spirit, dwelling on the edge of an upcoming thrill. The sexual pleasures came to a resounding pitch and then relaxed into a feeling that whatever happened was totally fine.

Curiously, they did not become pregnant that month. This only served to humble them, to suggest to them that conception was beyond their wildest dreams, intentions, and premonitions. Several months later, however, they did become pregnant. Lisa felt it as a twinge that raced up from her womb, through her solar plexus, and into her heart, like a determined "that's it." Rob didn't feel anything distinct until one week later, when he found himself utterly content, "like a contented cow," as he put it. Both their bodies had a subtle buzzing, which they had heard many months before, but it felt as though it was coming from every cell. During the months that followed they described two levels to the pregnancy: the throbbing internal gestation and its magnetic, nest-building effect on their home and relationship.

In the numerous experiences that accrue through such repeated ars erotica exchanges while following the passions of fertility, the possibility for innocent, sahaja or spontaneous conception—neither intended and planned nor unintended and accidental—can occur. What can be said about this event that is beyond the probabilities of any fertility calculations, any hopes, avoidances, or fears of conception, any thoughts or plans? I suggest the following: in some unfathomable depths a rhythm of destiny awaits the synchronous and choiceless touch of our human hands.

PROCREATION AND
THE SHARED-GENDER MYSTERY

The shared-gender mystery is nowhere more obvious than in procreative sexuality, for we see that egg and sperm require each other and that no woman ever became a mother without simultaneously a man becoming a father, technological interventions notwithstanding. Women and men confer parenthood on each other—with the help of the child, of course.

What obstetrician Thomas Verny, author of *The Secret Life of the Unborn Child,* and others have revealed and conjectured concerning the psychic relationship between a mother and the unborn child's "secret life" must be extended to include, equally but more subtly, the psychic role of fathers. Just as fathers have been invited into the delivery room only recently, our map of procreativity must restore them more fully into the whole of gestation.

Perhaps the loss of truly felt access to this psychic level of procreative rapport has contributed to our sense of pregnancy as being so difficult and isolating. We know in the biblical myth that the arising of a certain type of desire in the archetypal couple resulted in difficulties between the sexes and laborious childbearing processes. The breakdown of an erotically fulfilling sense of immediate rapport between the sexes may be an ancient and vexing story, yet through ars erotica sensitivities its recovery is within our reach.

Pregnancy might not necessarily get easier, but it might be experienced as more fully shared. As one of my interview couples stated, procreative sex was wonderfully different from conventional sex. It continued until the pregnancy test came back from the lab. They enjoyed an unexpectedly mysterious connection for all those days, which has, upon the birth of their daughter, become a substantive part of their felt relationship with each other.

We cannot easily say how any of the stressfulness of pregnancy could be experienced by partners who consider their pregnancy as an equally, although differentially, shared phenomenon. The psychosomatic interactivity of two persons is a profound mystery. My most impressive clinical experience was with a couple whose emotional impasse with each other was resolved when they shared, for the first time, the buried grief of an abortion that had occurred approximately nine months before. Coincidentally (!) the wife was headed for a hysterectomy within the next weeks because she had endometriosis. After the tearful session in which this couple finally shared their grief, the wife's next gynecological exam revealed a complete remission of symptoms, and the surgery was canceled.

Relational worship practices (as described in chapter 10) during pregnancy can be a way to share the special wonder of gestation and family creation. Over and over, fear of what is expected is displaced by awe of what is possible, and separations are transformed into viyogic unions. Yet we must beware of demystified expectations that seek "the perfect conception and pregnancy," "the perfect parenting," or "the perfect child." We must beware of fearing that which is inherently awesome. Instead, follow a mystery, for anything is possible.

SHARING A HOME WITH MYSTERY

Adult fertility reaches from this world into the world yet unborn, while children reach out from the invisible world into this more visible one. The contact of all adults and all children is based on this natural reaching toward one another's different worlds. The child's admiration and trust of the big adult and the adult's protective and nurturing feelings toward the child constitute the mysterious allure of their relationship.

Early adolescence is not best described as a "sexually confusing time." It is a time of intimate contact with the inherently mysterious passions of an emerging fertility and the possibilities within ars erotica, should urdhvaretas be yogically cultivated. No amount of sex education or yogic education will ever explain away the sense of mystery as fertility and accompanying new bodily pleasures and attractions converge within the (pre)adolescent, nor should such a goal be attempted. Efforts to preserve the awe and wonder of those times would, however, be a worthy endeavor.

In yoga's ars erotica, learning the "facts of life" becomes the teenager's careful discernment of and respect for the nuances of fertility and capacities for love and pleasure within himself or herself, in a wide range of meditative, musical, and dance modes, especially of pranotthana (intensified pranic activity), the adolescent precursor to possible kundalini awakening. It is not limited to instructions to "be contraceptively responsible," "wait for the right person," or "have fun—but don't get (anyone) pregnant!" Celebrating and ritualizing the onset of puberty for each child might prove to be an emotionally rich family event, as Julie, twenty-five, recounts:

When I was twelve, I had my first period, and we had this special dinner with my family, for me. My mother gave me six red roses and six white ones. My father gave me a pendant, which I still wear, with an infinity sign with two pearls in it. The pearls were like two souls meeting. My brother, I guess he was fifteen, gave me one of his bronze baby shoes. Two years earlier, I had given him a journaling book for his passage.

Over the years, this has had a great effect on me. I always can feel that world of fertility, passion, and magic, and it always adds something that I can share with just a few of my girlfriends and guys that I have been with.

Such are the ways of the passions of innocence in a family following a mystery, supportive of any future erotic pathway that one might choose. Tantric brahmacharya will, however, lose its allure if it is converted into a parental imposition that offspring "must follow."

Childless couples and individuals can assess what it takes in energy, resources, and maturational challenges to raise two or more children and apply "that amount" of creativity to their life projects. To grow spiritually, life itself is our gold standard for "what it takes" to become spiritually mature, whether for the lifelong brahmacharya yogi or the childless couple. Leading a quiet and happy life is another great achievement, of course.

ARS EROTICA FACTS OF LIFE FOR TEENAGERS

This section is for teenagers. Of course, there is nothing here that your parents or elders can't read, but it is intended specifically for you if you are in that time of your life. Indeed, due to high percentages of divorce, the early death of a spouse or other reasons, many middle-aged parents and even grandparents are now back into the dating scene that you approach or are currently in, for the first time.

Anyone can see that many adults are confused about sex and romantic relationships. In relation to you, they worry about the right things to do so you won't become sexually repressed, but they also hope that you can tell the difference between love and sexual attraction and won't seek out porn sites, while telling you that sex is a normal part of life. They worry that you will get HIV or herpes. They fear that you will have babies by accident or that after you are older you won't have any, that you will get all hung up on "boys" or "girls" and you won't finish your education. Or that you'll get interested in the wrong kids, period. And, sadly, lifelong love and marriage is a topic that has much of the modern world quite baffled. Your parents might have immigrated to America from a culture with far less overt sexuality and are trying to attune you to the customs "back home."

You know it all by now, all the things that parents and other adults worry about when they think about sexuality. It's not their fault. They really have no alternative. The only choice they have is to be either hip parents or firm parents—or some combination of the two. I assume that everyone is trying to do the best they can, parents included. I'd just like to share another approach to sex with you.

There isn't even an English word for what I want you to think about, so I'll use the one that comes from India, brahmacharya (pronounced: bra-ma-char-ee-ya). It means a way to live to know your absolute potential through your own experience of your mind and body and your relationships with others.

This is where meditation and yoga come in. Meditation can give you a sense of satisfaction that is all your own, that no one and no thing can take away. Brahmacharya gives your meditation the best fuel imaginable: your young-adult energy. Yoga exercises work like a nuclear reactor to convert this energy into potent forces that fill and nourish you. So brahmacharya means that you meditate and do yoga and breathing exercises instead of letting your energy out in sex (including masturbation). I will share some practices especially for teenagers in this section and you can draw from all the practices in this book and take some yoga classes, if you haven't already.

But consider from the very beginning that yoga is more than healthy exercises. It is based in a theory of human development that leads to the heroic heights of Buddha, Mahatma Gandhi, the Dalai Lama, and a couple you might not have heard about, known as The Mother and Sri Aurobindo, and millions of others. The yoga practices help the puberty that initiated you into adolescence to mature far beyond anything in medical books or modern theories of sexuality. Supported by yoga, meditation, and the many nonsexual couples' practices in this book, this maturation process goes on for your whole life, a process called urdh-va-retas, urdhvaretas.

For thousands of years, yogis have said the pleasures of yoga and meditation that include brahmacharya also go far beyond those of any drug out there. Indeed, all street drugs are poor copies of the real thing, known as rasas, the body's hormones of ecstasy that naturally emerge within the yogic lifestyle of a few hours of yoga and meditation before school each day. Ah, this will quickly lead to being asleep before 10 p.m., most every night.

While such a lifestyle is not necessarily in harmony with party and other late-night schedules, it will attune you to the great solar rhythms by which all life on the planet grows in harmony with the universe. I suggest that you try it for six months and see for yourself what it feels like. Even if you end your brahmacharya lifestyle after that, the memories will be with you, and the growth. Or you just might like it very much and your friends might, too. You could create your own circle, known as "Inner Heat Yogis" or some name you all create together. The movie about Saint Francis, *Brother Sun, Sister Moon*, tells the story of such a circle of young people in medieval times in Europe who followed a kind of Christian brahmacharya together. The Keanu Reeves movie *Little Buddha* also has some inspiring glimpses of one of the greatest, most mature of brahmacharins of all times, Buddha (not so much Mr. Reeves, as far as I know).

If you are going out with someone, there are plenty of nonsexual ways to get close to that person through brahmacharya. The relational worship practices described in this book can be as rewarding for teenagers as they are for adults. Just know that they are not meant to be a "come-on" to sex. Some of them are more emotional, and others are more physical. The key is to learn how to share your feelings for each other with these exercises, with dancing, singing, and meditating together. And, you don't have to figure out your "sexual orientation" in urdhvaretas, if you happen to be concerned about that. Let yoga and all these activities become your primary "orientation." For a while, just be a "brahmacharya yogi."

If you are not involved with anyone, you can do many of the practices alone. You might like reading the section in chapter 13 on solo urdhvaretas, too. Should you continue with brahmacharya for many years, it can give you a deep calm and serve as a basis for natural, higher states of consciousness. Drugs imitate these states, but they are illegal, and some are very dangerous. Yoga is not illegal or dangerous; it works with your own energies. It may be slower and less dramatic, but it will eventually exceed any chemically induced experiences.

Here are a couple of simple exercises to try out in a quiet place indoors or outside where you won't be interrupted for an hour or so. Sit comfortably in a cross-legged position for a few moments, then begin each practice.

YOURSELF BREATHING

1. This is easy. Each time you breathe in, say your first name or your nickname. When you breathe out, say your last name. Say everything very, very slowly during the whole time you breathe in or out. So breathing in, you might say your first name like this: RRRRRROOOOOGGGGGGGGGGGEEEERRRRRR or LLLLLLIIIIIIIIIINNNNNNNNNNDDDDDDDDAAAAAAA. Feel how unique you are, that there is only one you in the entire universe and there will always be just one you in the entire universe. Let the sound of your name go through your whole body and feel and appreciate your whole being. Start with ten minutes, then increase to twenty minutes.

2. You can do this alone or with a friend. With someone else, you can say each other's name aloud slowly to each other as you inhale, then things that you feel about each other, slowly, very slowly, as you exhale. Just feel what it is like. You can hold hands when you do this, and you will feel an electrical current flowing between the two of you. The current is the energy of your relationship, and you can feel it coursing all through your bodies.

3. If you want to feel this energy quickly by yourself, just shake both your hands vigorously at the wrist for twenty seconds, then stop and stir the tingle of one hand with a finger of your other hand by bringing it near but without touching it. Or have your partner stir your palm, without touching it, with his or her finger. You will feel the stirring on your open palm even though there is no physical contact.

4. If you are with your girlfriend or boyfriend and have sexual ideas about each other, just feel the feelings and breathe with those feelings while facing each other and holding hands. Just gaze at each other for two or three minutes, then close your eyes and be very still but relaxed in all your muscles. Any thoughts you

have will dissolve into sensations, and the sensations will be more pleasurable than the thoughts. In brahmacharya, you find out that not acting on them allows the desire to flow into the spinal pathway and diffuse throughout your body, leaving you feeling great.

ALTERNATE BREATHING

This breathing practice will help you discover meditation, which is your own mind and emotional heart before you get caught up in words and thoughts. By balancing the breath coming in each nostril, you balance both sides of your brain and the whole of your nervous system.

Sitting up straight, use your right hand to close and open one nostril at a time so that you can inhale and exhale alternately through the left and right nostrils like this: breathe in the left while the right is closed with your thumb; then breathe out of your right nostril while your fingers close the left. Then breathe in the right and out the left, in the left and out the right, and so forth. You can do the "Yourself Breathing" exercise at the same time, with each breath.

In this balanced condition, with your eyes closed, you can feel your own being, without any words. It is you, just you, directly. It feels great, and you can do it for ten or twenty minutes to relax or to prepare for schoolwork, sports, or almost any project. It centers you back into yourself, smoothing away any annoying distractions.

In brahmacharya you discover an essential feeling of love and understanding buried in each sexual desire and longing. You learn how to further sensitize yourself to the underlying creative forces in the universe. If you try this, you will see that sex is not just sex; it is the beginning of an enormous growth process, a big mystery that goes through many possible changes.

Of course, many people might tell you that you need sex to reach your potential. Certainly you can get an immense amount of value through sex, but it isn't necessary. You can always try sex, before or after you have tried brahmacharya. So you can do all the other things you like to do. Just remember these yogic teachings, follow them, and see what happens.

A few years of brahmacharya can begin to give you a basis of maturity for a lifelong, creative monogamous marriage where unconditional love, joyful sense of commitment and family life, and service to humanity can blossom. In such a union, the lovemaking spans from the playful and spontaneous to the devotional and profound, with the core being the 100 percent focus of the two partners upon one another. If you want to unlock these depths of eroticism—including the mind-orgasm of lifelong loyalty where your whole life "makes sense" in sharing it with someone who is sharing her or his life with you—it takes a regular yoga practice during your teenaged years till your midtwenties when this maturity begins to blossom.

From then on, for males, the pathway of endless erotic devotion becomes part of your sacred dedication shared with your partner without ejaculation's pleasure burst (except to coconceive with a beloved, for life). For females, I suggest you stay heart-centered, whether you seek the orgasm or not, since the female orgasm has only a feeling-connection to possible conception, and not so much a fertility-connection, as is the case with boys. While you are developing endless, heart-centered lovemaking in your twenties, thirties, and forties, contraceptives that you use should be considered as important training wheels, not as a permanent part of sex. Removing the training wheels requires complete confidence in your maturity together, gained via years of devotedly exploring the practices in this book and sheer fun of it all, known as lila, "play," in yoga!

Likewise, read and reread the "Retas Mysteries" section to develop ever greater respect for the profound fertility powers of ovulation and semen and for the creation of life itself. The sections ahead on "Inner Empathic Spaces" will help you connect more deeply with each other, and the "Communication Yoga" chapter will help you solve many problems that cause many couples to break up, including those with children. Keep learning together, and get help if you and your life partner come to a roadblock. You can both become so proficient in admiration, apology, and forgiveness, loving one another, missing one another, expressing deep gratitude, and fixing miscommunications that you will come to know unbreakable, unconditional love together that will last a lifetime, or two or more, in case you happen to believe in reincarnation.

8
Within the Intimus

*The Myriad Inner
Empathic Spaces (IES)*

Listening to thousands of couples describe their relationships, I came to believe that the vast majority live with each other in just a few of the myriad Inner Empathic Spaces (IES) that I will outline in this chapter. They know about some of these other rooms but can't get into them; instead they fight about "intimacy" and such things and thus end up spending lots of time in the basement that is the ball-and-chain marriage of late-night comedians and the fodder of divorce and its quite serious industries and consequences.

Of course, one room shared between two people who love each other very much will always feel "more than enough," but even couples who know this become amazed when inner spaces open up, such as "my glow of joy that triggers your glow of joy that then triggers your grabbing my hand that sends a throb of heat throughout my being that then sends a rush of tingles through you that bursts into the kiss that you give me that was triggered by your joy of my enjoyment of your joy of your enjoyment of my joy of my enjoyment of your joy . . ."

This is the realm of evanescent subtleties within the *intimus* (from the Latin word, meaning "within," "most interior") that are revealed by moment-to-moment, empathic meditative interactivity with each other:

"Two people chained to one another in endless causality/by their reverberating attractions to one another, endless irresistibility inciting endless irresistibility . . ."

Such joy and love will reverberate "positive patterns" *just as unstoppably* as complaints and frustrations reverberate negativity for couples who start out in love but get caught in patterns like "he said/she said," which then swirl into a downward sucking vortex of "well, fuck you for saying fuck you to me like you have done a hundred times in the past and I fucking ain't gonna take it any more"—the subterranean hell of a bad marriage, en route to legally carved-in-stone "Irreconcilable Differences and No Fault Divorces." Thus, heaven and hell aren't very far apart, though these two realms may seem "thousands of miles apart" to couples reverberating with each other "in hell."

The first experience of a new IES is like going into a room of your house that you have not gone into before and where modes of love are carried on and on that you might not have even thought possible, though you may have explored all sorts of scientia erotic fantasies of desire. It is right across the hall, yet only upon reaching this other room—the subjective experience of your lover—do you realize you have primarily lived your whole life until then in your own room, almost alone! But the power of "empathy" enables you to connect to others "in their own right," and even beyond the personal into transpersonal experiences of great mystery.

Such empathic connecting will immediately affect your partner to the degree he or she can feel, or is willing to acknowledge, your sense of intimate connection as "being real." While all kinds of superiority games, "I don't need you" games, "I am not going to forgive you for x, y, z this quickly" games, and so on get played in the space of "admitting/denying the feeling of positive connection," all sorts of ecstatic, playful, mind-and-soul melding games also can be shared in this space. The simple key to the latter is both partners saying, "Thank you" to each other for what each is receiving and let the sharing go forth. Thank you—gratitude—is all that most people really need to receive in order to go forward. Putting ever more *heart* into these words fills them with rasa, the creative seeds of warmth and encouragement.

And, there will be "rooms within this room" to further "reach into" that will awaken "new rooms" within oneself, which will then interact with all the rooms in your lover, in myriad ways, just as doubling the grains of rice from one square of a chessboard to the next will end up on square sixty-four with more grains of rice than exist on the entire earth. Thus: "My memory of the first time you looked at me is reverberating with how I feel now, ten years later, as you look at me. And that is reverberating with images of you looking at me this way ten years from now."

Both enter another room when one's partner responds with, "Your reverberating memories are deeply enriching my sense of the last ten years and my sense of the next ten years, too." And another room is entered with the next response of, "Thank you for thanking me for my sharing of that memory and that future projection. But right now your eyes are glowing like stars and the glow on your face has become so warm and loving that I must tell you, 'Wow, you are beautiful!'" When that is responded to with, "When you say I am beautiful, I suddenly feel very beautiful triggered by *your beautiful* love and appreciation of me! And suddenly *you* look beautiful in the very moment of telling me your compliment!"—then, wow, what a playground, far beyond cynical or demystified certainties that only *think* they represent the "*real* truths of love and marriage."*

I have aided thousands of couples to transform their rapport, merely by guiding them into these endlessly positive versions of their negative patterns. With all the saved energy, they can then apply sharing, giving, gratitude, forgiving, longing, creative problem solving, and even the powerful "X-rated" ars erotica spaces to catapult their marriage—the "same" relationship that once seemed "destined to fail"—toward *Sringara Rasa*, "Heaven Realm." So that you can also partake of such a transformation, here are sixty-four invitations to the spaces of IES.

---

*See Wittgenstein's *On Certainty,* on the whimsy that underlies many moments of "certainty."

SIXTY-FOUR INTIMATE SPACES
OF ARS EROTICA

Transforming Dialogue

1. A dialogue such as this—"Thank you for loving me," responded to with "Thank you for thanking me for loving you," responded with, "Thank you for thanking me for thanking you for loving me"—can sound pretty odd or Capra-esque corny, but couples who can attentively follow and participate in this back and forth repartee quickly get beyond cynical certainties and into the more wonderful life of the intimus. Indeed, for the hostile and love starved, sharing tears of gratitude will seem like the easiest miracle, yet one that most couples (and most couple therapies) have never tried. I recall a first session with a wife florid with rage at her husband's just-discovered affair, which closed in ninety minutes with them tearfully hugging and committing to a trust-rebuilding journey. Most Capra-esque of all was the Christmas knock at my door whereupon a trio of young daughters standing in front of parents whose marriage was similarly "saved" gave me a wrapped gift of a Shiva painting that hangs in my office with many other such mementos of successful grihastha therapies.

2. By staying within the intimus, your "endlessly reverberating positivities" can further awaken the retas-infused powers of the shared-gender mystery, the maturations that nourish the entheogenic rasa-chemistries of the great spinal charismatic awakenings of all times. Then, when issues arise, you will be entheogenically well nourished to respectfully discuss and resolve them.

    (This is in stark contrast to the couples who spend years swirling downward into the noxious chemistries of cynicism generating and fermenting ever more bitterly into their own, as well as their partner's, body—in therapy or on their own, at home—about who was right and who was wrong, who the bigger asshole, whose childhood trauma is messing up the other's life, who was the instigator of the affair, who will get the kids after the divorce on weekends or who will "never see these kids again!'" Entheogenic chemistries or diabolical chemistries? Not that hard to choose between them, and then to choose the former with a partner doing the same!)

Transforming Pleasure

3. Love as the range of wonderful, happy sensual pleasures one feels simply in one's own body from the touch of the other, at the level of sensation. Sheer pleasure has its limitations. A "for yourself" vibrator or male sex toy stimulates pleasure in its user but can hardly be said to "love" or "care about" the user or even "enjoy" being pressed against the user's body. Love, care, and the receiver's perceived enjoyment of the giver take place in another dimension, beyond but inclusive of sheer sensuality. Internet porn, likewise, may be extremely hot but does not care.

4. Love as the range of sensual pleasure one feels by tuning in to the textures of the skin of his or her partner's body. This dimension is the first to transit predominately outside one's own bodily focus. I ask a client to grasp the hand of his bitterly estranged spouse at a breakthrough moment, then ask, "How does her hand feel to you?" And he answers, "Kind and soft and lonely," whereupon tears well up in both, showing they have moved "in the unbearable lightness of being," from their dank basement into the sunroom of the quiet reunion.

5. The "rasa" taste of one's partner, being more internally perceived inside the mouth in a chemical reaction in the taste buds of the tongue, can feel deeper than sensual touch pleasure. I then ask that same couple, "Ah, giva kiss. . . . " And they do and glow with the fleeting radiance of their fragile, new life . . . to be nurtured and furthered and deepened.

6. Love as "feelings of closeness" that arise when you "reach your awareness" into the feelings that your partner is having, "over there."

> *In the Vedas two birds are on a branch,*
> *one eats,*
> *the other watches,*
> *feeding upon the eating one's sheer enjoyment,*

who enjoys the watcher's enjoyment of her enjoyed feeding,
adding to the other's adding to . . . .
The memory of it backward,
the looking forward to it again,
becoming other memories
inspiring other lookings forward
becoming other memories becoming other memories . . .
Everywhere you look,
then, now, later, feeding or being fed upon,
like the darting beam of a diamond-faceted miner's lamp,
love and nourishment are there and there and there,
as a mushrooming infinity of bliss.

The Power of Longing

Most couples love or feel into only the same few rooms, perhaps their whole lifetime, so they will always long for more. But longing must never be miscast as complaining. "I long for you" is beautiful, while, "Why can't you connect with me the way I want you to!" is shrill and disempowering all the way around. If you convert all complaints or frustrations into statements of "longing for," you will spare yourselves a lot of bitter anguish or rhetorical questions such as, "How could you!?" that have very little creativity in them. Longing has a wide array of velvety-rich tones:

7. Missing at a distance, over time.
8. Awaiting the return of symptom-free health during various severities of illness and caring for one another in the meantime. This, of course, is a vast realm of love, compassion, giving, receiving, gratitude for all, including having people in your life you want to care for this much.
9. End-of-life elder care is such an honor, if not also incredibly difficult and eventually beyond most any one person. How amazing love is . . .
10. Desiring and yearning for the look or touch or erotic heat or the very next moment or millimeter of closeness with one another.

11. Proustian closets and trunkfuls of wistfulness, memory-meandering sunsets of nostalgia from the ever-receding past (see Satyajit Ray's *Pather Panchali,* Song of the Little Road) for a cinematic masterpiece of such ars erotica themes).

12. Irreversible losses and heartfully grieving love for the dearly departed love-mate.

The Power of Reunion

Each of those rooms of longing has its own realms of satisfaction:

13. Reunions that come after a distancing miscommunication has been repaired.

14. Teasing playful, squealing reunions.

15. Unbridled, shirts-torn-off, mutually ravishing, "I can't wait any longer" reunions.

16. Unbelievable, long-lost and almost-given-up reunions.

17. Synchronistic, laced with mysterious coincidences reunions and dream visitations from those distant and living or long departed.

18. Predictable daily life reunions at the end of the day, upon simply waking next to one another for another day—by the grace of God.

19. Decades of past separation ended in deathbed reunions (common in long-estranged family relationships).

Becoming More than Delicious

20. Love as the range of sensual-emotional pleasures you feel as intensified arousals as a response to the pleasure your partner feels enjoying the texture of your body and the beginning of really getting into each other, physically.

> *With my eyes closed I feel you discovering more of your own*
>   *beauty*
> *as you feel me savoring you.*
> *In my mind I imagine being in your mind*
> *just as your taste is still on my lips, yours devouring me,*
> *your eyes now oblivious,*

you washing forth back like waves along a foamy darkened
coastline
everything fading backward receding into the ocean's ever-
shifting maw.
As if you had been breathing underwater for a long time,
you look up, your face now blurred with drunken passion.
I give up, you said. You are torturing me. Take me. Care of
me.
Then muffled tears lost fragments of rearising long-dashed
hopes.
You: I am delirious. Me: In a good way, I hope. You: Yes, in
a very good way.

21. This rasa-pleasure deepens in the experience of "being lusciously tasted as being more than delicious" by one's licking, sucking, kissing partner.

22. What a challenge to raise one's own identity to the space of being more than delicious to another person than one could ever have imagined!

23. Love expressions that feel as powerful as the drives of self-preservation and of breathing itself:

How far the sustained kiss?
The same breath shared mouth to surrendered mouth,
back and forth, over and over,
higher and higher
exceedingly relaxed exploring etheric realms
now become asphyxiating hungers voraciously aiming
where the life sparks in each other incept
pit of chest, core of brain.
Taking it no more, our minds silently explode with longings
electric,
soundlessly shriek, ungrasp the current us
squeeze another us breathless into There—
become a single throbbing, thadoom thadoom emerges,
the Universal Us swells in grandeur,

lungs stilled, minds now breathing directly into minds,
we collapse gasping amazed.

24. In so feeling yourself "being delicious" to your partner, your own body feels delicious to yourself. This causes deeper rasas and radiances of vitality, joy, and love to flow and intermingle with those of your partner and alchemically uplift each of you in their endlessly escalating reverberations. The shared-gender mystery awakens further.

25. Rasa-aphrodisiacs ("enhanced" oxytocin?) flowing through your veins and energies are traced to their flowing into another room in your own being that is your subtle (vibratory) body. When you become honey, mead, wine, soma-psychedelic to yourself and to your partner, who has also awakened the faith and belief and responsiveness to such ars erotica possibilities, then you will be *there,* in the subtle body mansion of many rooms.

The New World of Ars Erotica Spaces

26. Love as the range of sensual-emotional pleasures one feels in tuning in to the effect that your intensified arousal causes in your partner, whereby "the point of no return, edge of the flat-earth, genital-centric male scientia map" evaporates in the heart orgasms of endless devotion, mystery, exploration, new arousals, and entheogenic bodily awakenings. Going fully over the edge into this New World of ars erotica spaces, one also leaves behind scientia-tethered, "retention strategies" or perhaps even wondrous "multiple-orgasm pursuits."

27. Some people remain quiet or minimally moving in lovemaking and feel very close to each other.

28. Others pound and claw the bed in overwhelming physical passion, crying out to all gods and goddesses of devotional love.

29. Others spin into another and another position like a cascade of two tangling alleycats, or twined together like two snakes become one, breaking free of everything.

30. Others unfold yoga asanas, like mound-arching *chakra-asana* or

coccyx-heating *bhujanga-asana* cobra (see page 206).

31. Full-lotus *padma-asana* (see page 205) or *siddha-asana* (see page 206) might emerge out of the heat of passion, electrifying spines, lifting each of you off the ground, reaching for the sky, holding and holding the pose.

32. Breaking through one fear after another into the endless energies of rasa passions outside gravity of the flesh-body, completely beyond the fatigue of time and exhaustion.

33. Clothing torn off each other, due to completely irresistibly loved and adored bodies, now out of control and "beside oneself" (*ek-stasis*) with awe of the beloved.

34. Or dissolved in the melted-together closeness in the heart cave's warm sheltered stillness.

35. Or looking, they see the blush, the glossy eyes, the decades-shed mystery face, the self-biting of one's own lower lip in being over-whelmed by another.

36. Or laughing together like two raucous jungle parrots.

37. Or churning into one another, this way and that way, like wind-whipped ocean waves of honey.

38. Or crying together like two lost children clinging to the raft of life of each other, shivering with closeness, as if the only two humans on the planet.

39. Or meeting as a dream come true that wasn't supposed to be able to happen, but happened, all the same.

40. Or moaning under the burden of excessive oneness or whispered endless missives, "you, you, you, yes, yes, yes . . ."

41. Love as the range of sensual-emotional pleasure one feels in oneself after tuning into the new and higher level of arousal that you now feel, after sensing the increased arousal in your partner that was a response to your ardor. Wonder of wonders!

42. All the above, but now adding in your commitments to one another, through thick and thin, good times and bad . . . Lifelong loyal love: the endless, long-brewing entheogen!

43. Tuning in to your partner's pleasure as he retells favorite stories of your couplehood together, stories that seem to reach toward arche-

typal "universals" of all lovers of all times: the endless Shiva-Shakti dance!

44. Deep forgiveness that might suddenly emerge, as you both get beyond ordinary history of grievances, judgment, resentment, pettiness.

Reflecting Smiles

45. The joy of seeing your partner smile that causes you to smile. The dance of erotic intrigued smiles, eyes opened, half-opened, fully opened, head rolling this way, that way, hair spreading out radiantly, like spun gold silver ebony bronze, in the breezes of your smiles . . .

46. The joy of knowing his smile is about you, seeing you, your beauty, and how much he loves you. His knowing the same about you.

47. Knowing that your smile in seeing him smile at you will cause his smile to deepen into a blush of glowing beauty that your smile has caused. The world of blushing, a tumescence of the soul, is magic and holy, a holiness that embraces lust, love, and intimacy. It is the now-visible radiance of your soul that glows all around you. Couples realize that blushing is a climactic tumescence of the entire bloodstream, radiating mysteriously interactive feelings and rasas. Orgasms of sheer smiling emerge, orgasms of unstoppable laughter too. You share the liberating realms of "oh fuck!" profanities-as-wild-exclamation-points-of-overwhelm!!!!

48. Close your eyes and see the blush as memory, as inner blush, as inner smile, the soul's orgasm via minute after minute of heart-to-facial poignancies, tears streaming down faces.

Sharing Gratitude

49. Gratitude can be playfully, teasingly expressed to your partner for the gratitude he has expressed to you. "You made me love you this much! It's your fault!"

50. The depth of gratitude that comes only after you have expressed so many details of how your whole life has been enriched by your

partner that it takes you an hour (two, three) to tell her. Your chemistry of love brews ever-deeper feelings, as the fifth to tenth to sixtieth minutes stretch on and on in your stories of gratitude.

51. The fully entheogenic state of love, awe, and gratitude that comes through prolonged sharing, which you can only compare with profound peak or mystical experiences in temples or at the end of meditation retreats, at births, or journeying on sacred medicines or psychedelics.

52. Tears of joy and gratitude begin to flow down both of your cheeks. You find you have stopped breathing and feel beyond life and death. Some become delirious; what is known as *murcha* and *vyutthana,* swooning and resurrecting, can occur.

Dimensions of Completion

53. Tune into and enjoy the dimension of giving the hug, and also the dimension of receiving the hug, and the "interactive dimension" where the hug "mingles" you together, toward an experience of shared love and completion into a wholeness of male and female together. Gender differences? No, gender-mystery sharing!

54. When you physically separate, you can notice that, emotionally, you are just as close as when you were hugging.

55. You can cherish this knowledge all day long, even if you are a thousand miles apart. Likewise, you can derive pleasures, smiles, blushes, erotic arousals, and wonderful memories when you imagine your partner, a thousand miles away, also experiencing pleasures, smiles, blushes, erotic arousals, and wonderful memories as he thinks about you! This is viyoga, the urdhvaretic heart-anguish-love-orgasms of separation.

56. Sometimes partners will both telephone one another at such moments and both get "busy signals" on their phones because they are calling each other at the exact same time!

57. You can create a Memory Altar in your bedroom with mementos such as photos, sentimental gifts, romantic travel souvenirs from various places, birthday and other celebrative cards, and so on. You can have a locked treasure box of "secrets" for special mementos, such as

buttons torn off from shirts or blouses in moments of irresistibility.

58. You can look at the Memory Altar together, or imagine your partner looking at it when he is alone in the bedroom. Or imagine you are being visualized from afar, as you reminisce and smile, pausing alone at your Memory Altar, and see your partner's smile in her, afar, visualizing you, which evokes a smile on your face that evokes a smile on her face . . . You will be experiencing the viyoga of infinite unions in physical separation, once you open the door of consciousness into this love-space beyond any distance.

Creating Family, Embracing the World

59. If you have children, you can marvel together that your shared love created new life, and see how your children visibly grow and change every day.

60. You can together marvel that you have "made" your four parents into grandparents and created unimaginable joy for them, who can now see their lineages growing into the future for many decades, even glimpsing the image of their great-grandchildren being born into the marriages of their grandchildren . . . and then glimpses of their great-great-grandchildren, ad infinitum!

61. Marry young, and you might see your great- and great-great-grandchildren! So you and your spouse can now imagine decades ahead (or years, or maybe it has already happened) when you will be grandparents together, as your children get married and have children, and decades more into the future when you become great-grandparents, and so on.

62. All the above can filter into your daily memories, smiles, touches, and hugs, cooking together, shopping together, driving in traffic jams together, and your ars erotica lovemaking; you can watch for even deeper blushes and smiles and sexual arousals and meaningful pineal orgasms of inner light and celestial sounds and endless vibrations and creative inspirations to save the world family.

63. When the pineal puberty emerges, all the preceding dimensions are uplifted, again and again, into a near permanent maturity of the entheogenic body-mind-soul.

64. You know to your very bone marrow that life is infinite and that love holds the universe together; you wonder whether the "make love, not war" passion of the sixties might be matured if billions of people were in creative "till death do us part" ars erotica romantic relationships, making it powerful enough to actually manifest a "One World Family" peace.

I arbitrarily stop at sixty-four, but I could go on and on, endlessly, and never tire of it, nor would you! Indeed, exploring these transforming possibilities indicates that the 50 percent divorce rate is the outcome of a massive scientia sexualis lack of ars erotica seed-within-seed-within-seed imagination and sharing.

9

Communication Yoga

Verbal intercourse is the process of coming to understandings: the first words exchanged by intrigued strangers at a party; the auspicious closing words of a first real date; the first fight and all further difficult and passionate communications of apology, forgiveness, accusation, demands, ultimatums, confessions, and resolution; the heightened moments of avowal, gratitude, praise; the innocence of kidding and playing; poetic characterizations of love; proposals to live together, marry, conceive a child, separate, end separation. Such are the more momentous erotic communications, each generating a unique spectrum of emotions, orgasms, possibilities, and mysteries.

As an erotic medium, language is alive with suggestiveness, and even our most black-and-white statements are replete with innuendos, mutability, and implication. All take place in time, thus all bloom and wither in evanescent emotional subtleties. Within the domains of mystery, verbal communication must honor what cannot be said at the present time, what remains implied and ambiguous—between the lines, cleavages, and passages of language itself.

In support of the current psychological interest in clear and direct communication skills, I add my concern for the subtler aspects of nuance, the inscrutable but irrepressible value of the unspoken and untranslatable textures of different silences and gestures. Both precisely hewn clarity and unspeakable poignancy have their place in spoken passion. Indeed, we might benefit from learning a few dozen Sanskrit, French, Russian, Swahili, and other words to express what English cannot easily convey.

What lives in poignancy flickers within the impossible becoming possible, like a child's first steps, like the profusely meaningful warbling in one's voice while proposing marriage or the rise of one's anger already softening before the contrition in the eyes of the accused. The openness of our perception and the living responsiveness of the mercurial perceived are always at stake, for what we miss in any moment shrinks our world into one of ever-grosser generalizations and lifeless approximations. We must remain meditatively sensitive to the flowering of emotional subtleties that rectify the past, moment to moment. An ear tuned to mystery reveals innuendos of apology for the harm done in every sarcasm, nuances of trepid hope to be accepted in each defensive remark, a backhanded well-wishing in each shaming slur—in the other's or our own voice.

To the "lower state of consciousness" of cynical certainties or even well-intended demystified certainties, negative patterns of communication can seem like carved-in-stone roads to divorce. However, as Einstein noted, the world's intractable problems ("negative patterns") cannot be solved while in the same state of consciousness in which those problems arose. The synthetic approximates of the rasas provided by medicine have shown us the power of "state changing chemicals," but rasas are infinitely better.* Sharing five to ten minutes of extended compliments and expressions of gratitude brings about entheogenic states of consciousness wherein numerous problems and negative patterns can be creatively addressed. Without such an orientation, ordinary logistics and complaining of woes will tend to take up most of the "air time" of your communication with one another; that is, most of your whole life. Becoming sentimental in simple ways with urdhvaretas is the path to lifelong love and awakening.

---

*Indeed, I have helped many suicidal or psychotic folks uplift themselves via intensive complimenting over the course of several months or years, including those who, for a time, benefitted from the security of a hospital setting. For more, see Sovatsky, "Clinical Forms of Love Inspired by Meher Baba's Mast Work."

The first social steps into urdhvaretas for any of us are no further away than the simple graciousness manifested every time we:

- Thank or admire someone instead of taking it all for granted
- Listen empathically, instead of self-centeredly reacting to the other's words from our ego
- Deeply miss someone to the point of feeling connected to them, instead of blanking out or resenting the time apart
- Apologize or forgive self or other, instead of cultivating grudges or self-loathing
- Develop equipoise to channel our frustrations and angers toward creative solutions, even in the very moments of upset
- Honor close "seed relationships" with family and spouse or, if single, flirt with others but with the hopes of a lifetime

Thus, we become everyday urdhvaretas yogis and mature into ever more capable, ensouled-embodied persons.

TWENTY-ONE VERBAL ASANAS OF CREATIVE COMMUNICATION FOR COUPLES

I have created a list of twenty-one pointers based on my forty years' experience in transforming troubled relationships into creative ones. May the powers of retas that live within each point blossom for you and yours and may your love last forever.

1. To initiate the sharing of compliments, closely listen to one another with gratitude, so that the first thing you say is, "Thank you for telling me . . . " followed by a recounting of the key points your partner has made. Thanks can include gratitude for "being entrusted," for "the courage it took" to reveal certain thoughts and feelings. You can also extend your thanks with appreciation of the love for you that is implied.

2. Consider the positive implications of your partner's suggestions that go beyond his initial ideas. If there are points with which

you disagree, you can bring them up later. They won't get lost, but maybe they will become irrelevant. Adopt the goal of the "five minute compliment!" Imagine receiving the same type of enthusiasm; wouldn't you like it? Yes!

3. When the rasas of urdhvaretas awaken, then the all-day appreciations blossom, as partners go from simple "Thank you for saying that . . ." into endless details with their words of appreciation:

> *Thank you for sharing all the details of your life with me, thank you for being my love-partner for these many months, years, decades. Thank you for the beauty in your voice as you speak. Thank you for doing the daily hour commute to your office to support our family and to give the world your work. Thank you for caring for our children with love and always bringing the best to them, teaching them endlessly. Thank you for your concern for your parents and my parents that means so much to them and to me. Thank you for how beautiful you looked when I first met you and for how you look right now. I would like to play that song right now that says it all even better, "shower the people you love with love," and "more love, more joy . . ." and listen to it together with you while sharing Nyasa with you.*

4. The great secret of creating unbreakable love, beyond the "pull of gravity" toward too much moan-and-groan, lies in becoming aware of beautiful details and more beautiful associations from your whole life and putting all such thoughts into words together over and over again in the same or in new ways. Adding in the yoga ars erotica practices, especially Relational Worship practices and alternate nostril inner marriage breathing (see page 150) and the seed powers of urdhvaretas awakenings can uplift you into these joyous ways, even if you were divorce-bound a few months (or hours) ago.

5. Never mix "positives" and "negatives" in the same paragraph, much less the same sentence, as in: "You are being much more appreciative, *but* . . ." This practice alone will enhance your entheogenic feeding of one another to an amazing degree, as I have seen in thousands of couples. The heart opens and opens with positives

coming its way. Inserting a zinger into it might seem accurate or even funny but can trigger recoiling self-protections in the opened heart.

6. "May I share my concerns about your points now?" is a great way to switch to your counter-opinions, after hearing a "Yes, of course, I am all ears." The mind of your partner has prepared his heart for these counter-ideas by switching from heart-space subjectivity to more objective listening.

7. When we are in strong states of objective consciousness,* we are able to retain equipoise while hearing all sorts of criticism as "information," as "the experience of another person," as "extremely painful to another person," and even "as being believed to be caused by me (the objective listener)." In other words, the objective listener does not get "triggered"—a matter of subjective consciousness.

8. Such preparation and objectivity deserve more profound references such as "respecting one another," or "I-Thou-ing" one another. The easiest way to respect one another is to not mix positives and negatives in the same sentence or paragraph but to announce a "new paragraph" with a request as noted in 5.

9. The receiver of the request can say, "Thank you for preparing me to shift from my subjectivity to objectivity. In fact, I know you are trying to preserve our marriage by practicing this simple communication request, hoping to keep us together, loving our children and someday our grandchildren together, so I feel your deep partnership in preserving respect between us. I will always notice and hope to acknowledge this, for our sake and that of our children's children, as well as for the rest of tonight.

10. Retas, the seed forces that connect us with the origins and rarest maturities of life itself, invisibly permeate the mundanity of daily communications, especially hidden and lost for couples in periods of crisis, teetering in cynical certainties that can easily pile up and flip the switch to divorce, with fearful rasa-passions such as "I can't take

---

*Objective consciousness is a better name, in my opinion, for what other teachers refer to as "being nonjudgmental, being *really* present."

it any longer, I gotta get outa here!" Recovering retas depths during a crisis can revive the deeper purpose of your marriage and save it. Tapas, the passionate heat that emerges while straining within a dire situation toward its resolution can end up succeeding, as I saw with a therapy client couple, very much in love, but paradoxically stuck in bitterest acrimony for some eight years after an affair had been discovered. I had each partner, one at a time, hold a challenging standing pose until each started quivering and sweating as a "tapas" action of contrition and verified forgiveness, while the other one watched and winced until the watcher could not bear empathically feeling the strain of the tapas-pose holder. "Stop, come down from that pose! I feel your pain, I give you my deepest apology, once more!" Then, reversing roles, the other called out, "I am free of angers, come down from the pose, I forgive you!" The grateful Christmas cards I now get verify the longevity of their tapas breakthrough.

11. Ask sincere questions and learn to hear sincerity in each other's communication. This isn't as easy as it sounds, because of common moods of suspicion that make us greatly reduce our ability to grasp the sincerity of a question when beset by fears such as, "Why are you asking me this, do you think I am against you?" Even announcing, "I have a sincere question, may I ask you now?" is a great protection against the slippery slope of suspicion and ambiguity. Ambiguity of moods and evanescence of feelings can be part of the sliding down, while preparations will give you traction to hold your ground together. Complaints are really longings, stated in the negative. Restart your complaints as longings and couple them with suggestions of ways to experiment with sharing or satisfying these longings, rather than blatant outbursts. Should complaints pop out, we can later clean up with apologies and forgiveness for our "all-too-human" ways, followed with objective problem solving that aims into the future.

12. Labeling our frustrations "our real, authentic feelings" pertains only to the realm of cynical certainties. Adding "for now" to any declared frustration allows the future to breathe its openness into such so-called "real feelings."

13. Rhetorical sarcastic questions are like double black diamond ski slopes that can drop off into the abyss of cynicism, scoffing disrespect, demeaning feelings and facial expressions. A question such as "Why the hell did you do that?" implies "What an idiot you are, no matter what answer you choose to tell me, it will merely clarify for me the stupid nature of your reasoning process." If you are asked a sarcastic question but are able to deflate it to an objective inquiry and respond to that, it will have very powerful beneficial results.

14. Phrasings such as, "What were your objectives in doing it that way? What was your goal?" have a good chance of being heard as respectful inquiry, and if you are both working on your communication, it increases your chance for success.

15. The past is over. After a while of hassling over a bad thing that happened, switch to experiments to try next time.

16. Let the meaning of your words do the communicating and possible persuading, not the LOUDNESS of your voice. Let your reasons be stated as "good reasons" but not "the only reasons." Let your ideas be "possibilities" rather than "my-way-or-the-highway" ultimatums. Aim for dates rather than setting dates whenever possible.

17. Let your ultimatums have conditions to reverse them. Be committed to helping each other successfully achieve all conditions, ultimatums, requested changes, and so on. Be a team. Male and female power circulates better this way, rather than leaving us feeling cut off from half of the human universe (for gay or straight folks or those living in any of the many nuances of gender sharing).

18. Create the protocol that a hug asked for will always be given, even at very difficult "I don't feel like it" moments. Rasa of love and closeness can be renewed by such "Help! Hug Me" requests that recenter us for better communication five minutes later.

19. Reach your listening across the distance between the two of you into the subjectivity of your partner, feel it like a glowing light inside their heart, as he or she shares conversation with you.

20. Even if you have angry reactions and your own hurt feelings to express, tune in to and develop the equipoise of forbearance; wait till your thank-yous are complete before sharing your subjective

responses. Upsets of all sorts can almost always wait till then. Emotional mastery can come to displace "spontaneity" and reveal poignant feelings of empathy for others that make "spontaneity at any cost" seem highly overvalued.

21. Whatever is shared falls into the vibratory, reverberating realm of the shared-gender mystery. Fights typically reverberate more fights, escalated in the panic and pain of falling further away from each other. Wonderful couples are thus, with ever-greater centrifugal forces, flung out of the intimus into the freezing outer orbits of cynical certainties where destructive actions like divorce seem to "make perfect sense." But as you both dedicate yourselves to extending your compliments and gratitude into five- to twenty-minute romantic treatises or poems, you will keep your relationship in the intimus.

The power of such interactions can result in transformations that can seem almost surreal, such as when I have seen couples co-create a positive sharing (now embedded with "thank you," "you're welcome," "I heard you say," "I need a hug," "may I hug you?") from a conversation that twenty minutes before had bounced their escalating frustrations back and forth to a final sadomasochistic frenzy of, "I can't take your shit any longer, I want a fucking divorce!" "Good, fine, fuck you, I beat you to it!"

As you develop "ears of listening gratefully," and all the rest, you too can solve your problems carefully while staying in the intimus. Your poems of gratitude will pile up as memories that can reverberate into the present (just as complaints pile up for those who miss this simple but deep guidance, who then feel "trapped"); then, as the years go on, you share only "more love and more joy," as Smokey Robinson once lyricized. May all find their way to the intimus; it's right *here* and *here* and *here*.

10
Relational Worship

The primary word I-Thou can be spoken only with the whole being. Concentration and fusion into the whole being can never take place through my agency, nor can it ever take place without me. I become through my relation to the Thou; as I become I, I say Thou.

All real living is meeting.

MARTIN BUBER, *I AND THOU*

The practices presented here will guide your exploration of your own deeper potential as individuals and as a couple. For couples who choose tantric brahmacharya for a period of time, they can be doorways to profound transformation.

In the early stages of brahmacharya relationship, love, commitment, and passion are expressed through feeling each other patiently, even confusingly, endeavoring to discover the urdhvaretic tonalities. For what will be before you is not some perfected state of tantric nirvana but your utterly human partner entering, just as you yourself are, an unknown erotic world, while the more familiar one might still be sending beckoning images. We become partners in this most uncommon and uncharted exploration, perhaps also sharing how little we actually know about erotic mystery rather than how much skill and prowess we have.

That is, we engage in a sharing of innocence, wonder, creative powers, courage, and humility. Sexual thoughts, should they emerge, can seem to be a familiar refuge from the nakedly intimate contact that can blossom into spinal surges of radiant shuddering. The early weeks of practice, then, evince a naïve faith. This phase can be short. Appreciate it with the exploratory feel of a second adolescence.

Longings intensify and subside over and over again as various emotional peaks are released into these new tumescences of heart, breathless gasps, and eye-rolling trance-ecstasies. Your glands and nerves buzz with energy and arousal while, gradually, the ars erotica ardor of tapas initiates an internal alchemical process. As the weeks continue, the heightened energies are reabsorbed, allowing your glands and cells to be nourished by this enhanced essence. You are getting "hot and bothered," and it doesn't go away. Instead you are being moved, danced this way, then that way, played by an inner oceanic symphony. You are birthing your ars erotica body. As weeks become months, your glandular arousals will be slightly more fulfilling, charged up, or entheogenically active than previously. At this incrementally "higher" level of baseline functioning, these newly produced essences will be even more charged than the last, to be raised infinitesimally higher in the months to come. This is urdhvaretas. And as ars erotica, we have no problem including couples practices for a wide range of seekers in the same book that guides solo, inwardly married, "celibate" yogis. Profundity of pleasure is our compass, wherever it may lead us.

Over and over again, this hermetic, alchemical passion energizes lachrymose, salivary, genital, pineal, hypothalamus, and pituitary activity as well as the chakras and subtle energies. Psychologically, in the months and years to come, you will find that urdhvaretas satisfies you, fostering your ability to release the overgripping insecurity and under-gripping hopelessness of the teen-tethered genital primacy ego. That frees you to experience the rest of human development that has always awaited throughout the total expanse of the spine as anatomical-spiritual pathway.

Thus what follows are not mere instructions to be enacted or another set of erotic conventions to be performed and perfected. They are a set of structured suggestions designed to open up these ars erotica spaces. Mystery, subtlety, and discovery take precedence over formality and performance. In tantric brahmacharya, as in the infant's incarnating movements and in the hoped-for freedoms of conventional sexuality, there are no missionary positions to adhere to or rebel against.

THE GREAT GESTURE

1. Sitting opposite each other, hold hands so that right palms face down and left palms face up. This position is based on the tantric principle that energy enters us through the left hand and is transmitted out through the right.
2. Next, focus your gaze upon each other at the midpoint between the eyebrows. Continue to gaze at each other, going through various phases of recognition, mood, and attention.
3. Allow your focus to soften so that your vision becomes momentarily blurred, pulsing with your heartbeat. Then, very slowly, refocus. Do this periodically. It will allow your eye muscles to relax and to make possible subtle shifts of perception. Your partner's face will very likely change in appearance, perhaps seeming older or younger, more radiant, or filled with the impressions of past emotion and attitudes. You might also see a sense of his essence, a kind of pervasive quality that permeates all his aspects and actions. In these pulsings, vision reveals a living world. This relaxed vision is an early stage of pratyahara, gathered focus.

Try to find a balance point where you are equally aware of your own presence and the presence of your partner. As you come to hovering at this point of equal internal and external awareness, you will likely feel a kind of spacious opening occur, even a sense of timelessness. Your partner might appear profoundly unique to you in a curiously unsuspected way. As one husband said during his very first try, "I realized for the first time that my wife was giving me the love that I had always been looking for. I had never looked at her this long before." As the Krishna-kavi-bhakta George Harrison sang about such seeing, "Lulling me with those raincloud eyes . . . Melting my heart away."[1]

It becomes clear, as time passes, that you are each reflecting in your responsive countenance the image of beholding the other. You feel you have known each other for an indeterminate amount of time, perhaps forever. You experience yourselves as the same. You see a deepening beautification surface from each other's depths into the skin, eyes, and spirit, and it seems that this emerging beauty is the living response to your every willingness to see it. Let's call this "perceptual tumescence" or "visual intercourse," aiming toward shambhavi mudra, the puberty of the eyes and spiritual seeing. Much of what you see that moves you so is your partner's response to you, creating a kind of natural biofeedback that deepens intimacy. The beautification of each other feels to be endless and moving to ever more profound levels of assessment. Early dharana, as the sense of visual-emotional, mutual synchronicity, flutters.

Drink your partner in, taste him entheogenically through your eyes and pores. Each time you lower your eyelids, feel the caressing of his essence with your eyelashes. You will see his eyes moisten ever so slightly with ars erotica secretions of the heart's tumescence. Look with your heart and see that the varieties of tears are legion, revealing a whole expansive world of meanings and submeanings in every glistening radiance. If vision is through tears, which refract the entering light with a prismatic effect, who is to decide whether the dancing rainbows we see are best described as miraculous wonderments or merely as a peripheral and insignificant scientific property of optics?

The tumescences of shyness and blushing might also emerge, overcoming you with blue-pink whispers of unbearable beauty. For shyness always heralds a greater sense of being seen and known, of seeing and feeling someone seeing and feeling us. We blush in catching another seeing us, for shyness is the innocence that consecrates each birth and revelation of the soul. Shyness is not a problem; it is a precarious mystery tenderly shared.

Perhaps a tear will streak down your cheek, and you realize how much there is to you and your partner, how responsively connected you are to each other. Other tears might follow, yet you feel only momentarily melancholic, then joyous, embarrassed, then wholly softened, for these are the living tears of the "inner adult" of anahata chakra. If pains and angers from the past emerge, see them waver, like desert mirages, and then dissolve into the inestimable passions of virya, leaving you in the ever-forgiving vividness of the evanescent present-future.

In the togetherness now, the experience called "Sharing This" emerges. Such "suchness" is the furthering of dharana, revealing the near-unbroken flow of mutually absorbed contact. Couples feel, "We are really in it together!"

Perhaps the stirrings in your genitals, abdomen, heart, and throat, which mount, subside, and shift, now swell into your heart and throat. A subtle salivation, perhaps of a sweetened taste, hints its way into your mouth. In your unguarded state, it seeps out of the corners. You feel utterly innocent and uncontrolled, and your partner appears the same way, in the spell of bodily transformations. Did you know that the heart can "cum?" Now you do . . .

An undisguised openness and steady receptivity begin to unfurl, as heavy and unruffled as a warm flow of sacred oils. A breathless moment. A ringing silence. You both slowly close your eyes. Darkness. One psyche or soul. An ever-growing brightness dawns.

Throughout your whole body an inward caress causes you to quiver, then shudder; mystics have called this "the inward touch of the divine." Dharana, silence, dhyana. Billowing essence of boundaryless love here, there, everywhere. A sound, a smooth sound—breathing; one blood-stream, one pulsebeat, one passageway in: mother-father birth; the in-between; and then, out. Sounds of breathing in and out. The slow pulsing of the universe.

Your sighs of intimacy have now become deeply appreciative. You feel a tingling pass between the palms of your held hands. It traces up your left arm, into your throat, and down into your heart, abdomen, genitals, and spinal base. You begin to experience the subtle body channels, energies, and chakras. You can feel the spontaneous movement of urdhvaretas passion sending currents of pleasure throughout the internal musculature of your body, triggering the bandhas and various mudras, as tumescences, as puberties. You experience having a human body as a kind of fortuitous stroke of genius on someone's part, while the buoyancy of ars erotica attraction to the world around you feels as light and responsive as a feather.

Serenely still, your breathing suspends. Time withers, place evaporates. Kundalini-shakti stirs. Heat grows stronger within muladhara, your throat, your heart, in ajna between the eyes, in the midbrain area. Effortlessly, your tongue weaves back into your throat. A glow of electrical heat quivers, connecting the root of your tongue, throat, heart, spine, and perineum. A space of light opens. Time and more time, all is just time. The words pass, it's time, it's time.

You open your eyes slowly to a world of brilliance; the heavy-laden vineyards of the spirit have ripened. The entheogenic rasas are blossoming . . .

> A fountain of gardens, a well of living waters, and streams from Lebanon.
>
> Awake, O north wind; and come, thou south; blow upon my garden, that the spices thereof may flow out. Let my beloved come into his garden, and eat his pleasant fruits.
>
> SONG OF SOLOMON 4:15–16

You rest into each other's arms, feeling the heat and energy that is within and between you. Sitting up, you meditate quietly for an indeterminate time, then separate palms and smile, perhaps with some shyness.

NYASA

In Nyasa, touch enters the concentration of pratyahara and the mood of bhakti, devotional reverence. The subtleties of energetic transfer give it an urdhvaretic gist. You will need a vial of scented oil, not for massage or lubrication but as an ars erotica anointment. It should be special oil; if not, the practice of Nyasa will cause it to become special, for Nyasa is empowerment through touch, a kind of gender awe or worship.

1. Decide who will anoint whom first. Apply some oil to the middle two fingers of each of your right hands. Sitting across from each other, establish contact through gazing.
2. As the romantic subtleties of pratyahara emerge, slowly begin to raise your

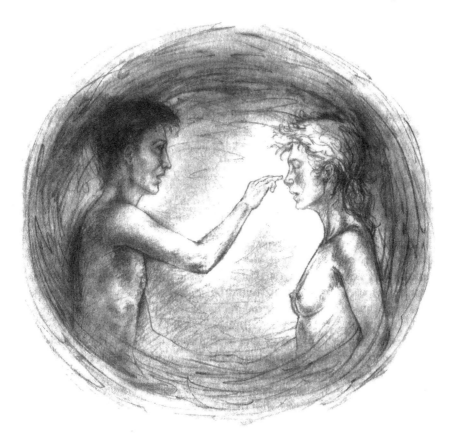

Nyasa

right hand—indeed, feel it tumesce—in synchrony with the slow passion of your inhalations, as if the breath itself raises hand and arm, body, gaze, and all toward the ajna chakra in the center of your partner's forehead. If breath should fill, pause; then, exhaling, continue the movement. Continue in this way so slowly that perhaps ten minutes pass before you have neared your partner's forehead. Let the awe of approaching a demigod or demigoddess slow you down. Each moment carries another degree of closeness, awe, and arousal and is unique. All else has faded into the periphery. Your partner's forehead opens even more, and wisps of energy flit out of its labyrinthian depths. Dharana glimmers.

3. You come closer and closer until the very radiance of your fingers can be felt by your partner, whose midbrow now palpably throbs, even glistens. Within inches, another microworld opens up. As in time-lapse photography of an unfurling

rose, duration dissolves like salt in the oceans. It just happens. Contact is made, and a wholeness of selves responds; bodies enliven, chakras whirl, koshas harmonize, retas distillates quicken.

4. Contact continues, essences mix together; the mystery of endless commitment, of following a forever mystery, surfaces. Eyes close. Opinions dissolve; marriage, no longer an "institution," choice, or task, becomes a living verb, a marrying, commingling of the two; the shared-gender mystery becomes an ars erotica condition of reverence that you now swim in together as your whole relational world, your reality that only spellbinds you further, absorbs you ever more into this new, vast realm of the intimus; dharana and dhyana glimmer; samadhi hovers in the far distance. Did you know that the pineal can "cum?" Now you do, as its entheogenic puberty quickens more and more over the months, years, and decades ahead.

5. Your hand lowers in synchrony with your exhalation until it nears your partner's throat, where the mystery of breath and pulse throb mysteriously. You finally touch just above the notch of the collarbone, where the windpipe recedes into the neck to carry the life air inward. Another world, different in time (for "time" has passed, "then" is invisibly gone) and being (for vishuddha now shows us other qualities of being) emerges. Other radiances, nectars, subtle hopes, and intimacies spark. Inspiration renews itself, the birth of words from ineffable missives.

6. Release. Lower your hand all the way and preserve eye contact until you feel like closing your eyes to follow the mystery, intuitively bypassing visual perception completely. Let your lungs "cum" with prana and surge into rapid, rapid, or . . . suspended . . . breathing. As you open your eyes, exchange the roles of anointer and anointed.

Although Nyasa can empower any of the chakras, the sublimative passion does not prefer svadhisthana as being more erotic than others merely because that chakra is associated with genital arousal. Each chakra has its own characteristic tonality of passion and energy. At certain points it may be unclear who is the initiator of this movement, the anointer or the anointed. Doing this practice with eyes closed creates another sort of spatial context through reaching out to touch the anointed.

MYSTERY OF BALANCE

1. Sitting cross-legged or in chairs, knee to knee, facing each other, join hands and raise your arms straight up, balancing their weight. Relax all other muscles and focus gently and steadily on your partner at ajna. As your arms get heavier and heavier, notice all the compelling questions you have about what you think you should do, what you think it means to your partner, what you think your partner wants you to do about it, what your proper roles are, and so on.

   What is maleness, femaleness, my needs or yours, caretaking, loving too much? What is commitment? All the popular "certainties" that circulate in the great anonymous now circulate in your own mind. Yet the weight continues, even if you cry or yell, "How much longer?" The fight last night or ten years ago, the little irritations of each other, like flotsam, float through your mind. None of these tirades, diagnoses, or "feelings gotten in touch with" help for long. In fact, they seem to separate you from something else: what is happening wordlessly, looking and straining and wondering, between the two of you now. *That* is an erotic mystery unfolding.

2. As you just share the weight, reaching ever more passionately upward, you find the balance. Mysteriously, the weight is gone. On and on the weightlessness of your arms continues, wavers, then returns for five minutes, or perhaps fifteen, twenty, a half hour, or longer. No complaints, criticisms, just the sharing of a difficulty that has, mysteriously, become something profound. Such sharing cannot be explained easily. Your inner adult emerges and grows in faith; the pains of your earlier years, no longer mere wounds, reveal their dignities (as you marvel at the subtle energetics and yogic processes just beneath the obvious, involving the early subtleties of virya). You dwell near ananda-maya kosha, beyond gravity's heavy pull.

3. You lower your arms and roll your eyes in astonishment, for your sharing of the difficulty has transformed it. Perhaps on the first try the transformation is wavering, or barely perceptible, but each try will have interesting results. This curious balance is not a goal; it is an inexplicable side effect of mystery shared.

4. You can use a timer to set the duration of this practice if you wish. Without a timer, another possibility avails.

The mystery of balance can also be explored in a group, with members seated in a circle, shoulder to shoulder and all facing the center.

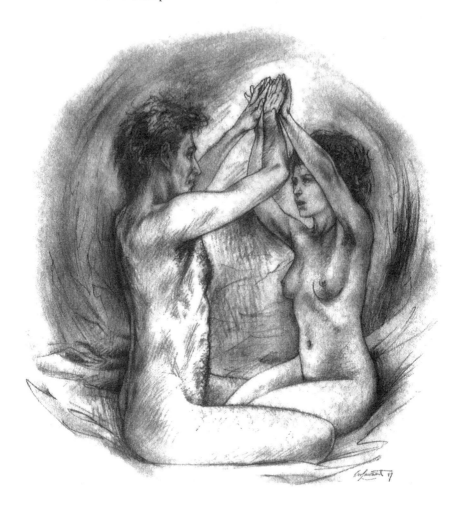

Mystery of Balance

Then, each joins hands with their neighbors to the left and right and all raise up their arms together with everyone gazing at the others around the circle. The power of the group can often be even more mysterious than that of the couple. Members feel the collective involvement as a sense of loyalty, brother-, or sisterhood. The group's purposes and struggles feel shared and uplifting for each individual who is having the same weightiness bearing down on her.

PRANIC MIRRORING

1. In this practice, you and your partner mirror each other's movements as you share a slow-motion practice of yoga asanas, synchronizing breath with movement. Taking three to five minutes, you might slowly reach across the space to touch hands or perhaps to exchange a rose or a gift.
2. Integrate pratyahara and dharana concentrations into the practice as well.

Dancing, of course, is a perfect activity in which to enjoy various permutations of pranic mirroring. Ecstatic dancing and Sufi whirling are well-known versions of passionate ars erotica dancing. Perhaps the energies will strongly awaken from within and "dance" you, as has occurred in charismatic spirituality worldwide, throughout all history. Should the esoteric belly dance of the ecstatic trance get activated, you will see how most scientia, entertainment-for-an-audience forms can inhibit the esoteric ars erotica powers from emerging. As Axis Mundi belly dancer Catherine Calderone said about her inspired undulations, "I would fall to the floor after an hour, exhausted from being danced by the Mother chanting and drumming, but then my body would get itself up again and again, undulating and swirling beyond myself."

THE SINGULAR ARS EROTICA KISS

Tantric brahmacharya can appear rather predetermined, especially in the first weeks of practice. The single kiss is an example of bringing an ordinary erotic gesture into the context of urdhvaretas. In conventional sexuality, the genital orgasm is the final gesture of erotic exchange. It is a way of dealing with the endlessness of erotic mystery within the driving currents of desire. That is the temporal function of the orgasm: to bring sex to an obvious and climactic close.

1. A single kiss can seal the meaning of a moment, for that is what is being called for when eros reaches this pitch: a sign, a ritual, a mudra, or a gesture that expresses what words cannot say.

2. Then, as this singular communication is completed, we allow the mind of the heart to absorb what has just been "said." Usually, we go on seeking more and more arousal through the enactment of escalating desires. In tantric urdhvaretas, we find another sort of erotic "more" in the meditative depth of the single kiss. Did you know that lips could "cum?" Now you do . . .

Remember the first kiss of a relationship? There is nothing to compare it to, and there never will be. There is a whole world of erotic meaning, value, and experience that comes from honoring and preserving the innocence and mystery that is revealed at such times. The first kiss, the singular embrace, deprived of a second, drops our hunger into the chasms of mystery. The eros of nonattachment and subtlety dawns. And then there are the rare ars erotica mystical kisses whose entheogenic powers uplift us to the heights of saints and enlightened beings of all times:

At nineteen years of age, Meher Baba (nee Merwam Sheriar Irani, 1894–1969) received a kiss on his forehead from the highly venerated Muslim woman, Hazrat Babajan (alleged to be 122 years old at the time), and then kissed her hands. That evening, he entered an altered state of blissful, "electrified" consciousness wherein he did not sleep for nine months. "I had no consciousness of my body, or of anything else. I roamed about taking no food . . . [and experienced] Divine Bliss."[2]

For the next seven years, he remained in a spiritual beatitude, beyond the reach of doctors and only gradually regaining ordinary capacities, but conveying to many around him various saintly attributes for the rest of his life. He remained in silence after 1925, made several teaching tours throughout Europe and America, and attracted a following of many hundreds of thousands worldwide who believed him to be an avatar, the most mature of saints in the Indian terminology.[3]

BREATHING MYSTERY

1. After establishing meditative eye contact, or after the Great Gesture or Nyasa, allow the feelings of urdhvaretic passion to become audible sighs. Sharing of these sighs leads to further sharing of them into greater subtleties rather than toward sex.

2. Allow the mystery of hearing each other's audible transmutation to affect you. This sets up an exchange of feeling that, over and over again, passes through the fires of urdhvaretas. The sighing may grow louder or softer or even into vaguely audible whispers; there is no singular direction, no specific crescendo to aim for.

 MANTRA CHANTING

According to the theory of mantra, specific sound vibrations have specific effects on various chakras and emotions. The mantras resonate and stimulate the chakras through this subtle vibrational massage. Melody and rhythm add two other common elements for erotic exchange, yet the medium is voices and feeling. Pratyahara and dharana emerge more easily when we have fed upon the sensations of mantra.

1. This practice can be engaged in alone, with a partner, or in larger groups with the use of instruments. The chanting can proceed at a steady tempo, or it can be carried away by the escalations of nearly unmanageable yearning into faster and wilder rhythms, at times surrendering even the formal mantras into laughing, crying, howling, sighing, and so forth.

2. Cycling from slow to faster and climactic tempos over the course of an hour or till dawn the next day can reveal a depth of passion that has earned bhakti yoga the reputation of being the most profoundly mysterious of yogas, unfolding the entire path to one who merely continues to surrender to its emotional depths. Even spontaneous dancing or impassioned pranayama and asanas can emerge. Thus, chanting is often called the nectar of devotion. The mantras *Ram, Om, Hari-om, Namo-Shivaya, Sita-Rama,* and *Om bhur bhuva swaha* are some possibilities. If chanting Hindu mantras feels too

foreign to you, the sound "ahhh" is in itself exhilarating. Did you know that your voice could "cum?" Now you do.

3. The spiritual side of mantra chanting as a devotional practice can also be explored. As such, the deity enters into the chanting (and the room).

RITUAL WORSHIP OF MYSTERY

The power of group ars erotica rituals underlies all of the world's charismatic religions. Indeed, the charismatic "divine gift" energies may trace back many millions of years in evolutionary history as being the primordial love-ins that uplifted prehumanity from mere "survival of the fittest" modes to "love one another" modes.*

Rituals reveal feelings of reverence, gratitude, honor, offering, and sanctity that many couples experience toward each other only during their marriage ceremony. Bringing these sentiments to mundane tasks can transform them into ars erotica intoxicating wines of devotion.

You can create fire, water, earth, and air rituals, group chanting and Nyasa practices, anniversary rituals, fertility rituals, menopause rituals, rituals for sharing the vows of brahmacharya, pregnancy, birth, and naming rituals, sunrise and sunset rituals, and home-building rituals. The use of symbolic ritual objects, gift giving, role reversals, and other dramatizations give our senses profound ars erotica stimulations, far beyond the surface desirability realm of the scientia sexualis.

---

*According to preeminent world historian William H. McNeill's *Keeping Together in Time,* "group rhythmic practices" (monkey-tribe log-tapping) may have created the first moods of Oneness in our prehominid ancestors millions of years ago. Intratribal anger was dissipated via drumming as the hormones of aggression transmuted or matured (or "evolved") into rasas of nascent collective devotional feelings. As these practices bestow great Darwinian "survival value," these tribes grew, while others that did not engage in shared "rhythmic practices" fragmented as aggression led to tribal breakdowns and divisions and lowered rates of group survival. Ah, the creative power of Om, Om, Om . . .

YONI-LINGAM WORSHIP

1. Consider the tantric ritual of meditatively pouring silver tureens of warm buttered milk over the top of a two-foot-tall, eight-inch-thick black yoni-lingam (a cosmic thallus set vertically into a cosmic elongated yoni base, itself extending laterally, funnel-like, over a foot from the lingam that is merged into its epicenter) and watching the creamy retas-rasa-milk pool into the creviced base of the yoni and overflow from its funneling end into another tureen set below.

2. As you pour and watch, repeat, "Om Shiva Shakti, Kundalini Ma!" over and over, as slowly as the buttered milk drips down Shiva and into Shakti Ma! Cast flower petals everywhere! Meanwhile, arrange it so that endless sitar music shimmers in the background.

3. Next, meditatively pour a tureen of sacred purple-red vermillion-dyed, warmed vegetable oil over the yoni-lingam, dripping blood-red down the lingam into the embracing yoni, mixing with the white milk still streaming down the side grooves and out. Sing "Kali Durgha, Namo Namah, Om Namo Shivaya, Om Namo Shivaya!" If you also jostle bronze finger cymbals twice, thrice, *zhing-zhing-zhing*, you will spread scintillations of awe into the air everywhere.

4. Then pour a tureen of orange-golden turmeric-dyed water over the lingam's top; watch as it mixes in the yoni grooves with the vermillion and milky swirling rasas from the last consecrations.

5. Then meditatively pour a tureen of white-clumped yogurt-water and observe how it slithers down the lingam into the awaiting yoni as you chant "Om Creators of the Universe . . . Om Oneness of the Two . . ."

Your dreams the next weeks will be Shiva-Shakti, retas-nourished, pineal-blossoming, whole-lifetime-awakened, within the cosmic ars erotica, far beyond anything known within the myopic Freudian herme-neutic and infinitely more expansive than the mere "Now." Indeed, the whole pretentious, "final word" claim of psychoanalysis of giving us the "one, real erotic truth" becomes irrelevant and distortive to our new ars erotica lives—an "invasion of the sacred," as my Indological colleagues call the "psychoanalytic gaze"—while "Now" is just the beginning . . .

A SUNRISE RITUAL

1. Wake up two hours before sunrise; bathe and dress each other.
2. Separate for forty-five minutes of individual yoga practices. Feel both the solitude and the longing for reunion.
3. Reunite at the specified time. Bow before each other. Share Nyasa and meditate together with the rising sun, beginning twenty minutes before sunrise. Feel the effects of the sun's slowly building energies.
4. Share the "Great Gesture" for some minutes after sunrise. Bow and thank each other and the day.

 ### SECRET KNOWLEDGE RITUAL

One of you is the initiate and the other is the initiator in explaining a new aspect of gender worship. The latter serves by teaching, and the former leads by being curious, and thus the mystery of shared power is revealed, even when it is made clear that one of you "knows" something that the other will learn.

The Tao Te Ching speaks of the "utmost mystery" as the close mesh between teacher and student, so intimate that an onlooker is unable to discern the roles.

 ### ONE-WORD RITUAL

In the "Great Gesture" take turns slowly expressing one word or phrase to each other, over and over, for example, "commitment," "yes," "love," "urdhvaretas," "I know only this," "together," "deeper," "more."

THIS AND THAT

This section includes an array of topics from diet, sleep, dusting yourself off after any "slips," and keeping your sense of humor, to a few words to sacerdotal celibates, guidance for a gradual celibacy, and the simplicity of a constantly worshipful mood.

Diet and Sleep

Since svadhisthana is also the taste center, some attention to diet can prove useful. Try a lighter diet, less spicy, in moderate portions, eaten earlier in the day, and leaning more toward vegetarian foods and away from heavy animal proteins. The lore of no garlic, onions, or mushrooms (too sexually stimulating, it is said) is worth experimenting with on an individual basis.

Sharing a pot of sage tea, skullcap tea, valerian root tea, or ginger and cinnamon tea is a soothing way to spend an evening telling brahmacharya stories around a campfire and will have a calming or balancing effect. But the effects of such practices must be considered as limited. Occasional fasting can provide a dual recovery of a balanced relationship with food and sexuality. Some yogis prescribe fasting for one day a week, merely to relax the digestive system. I suggest exploring and sampling what appeals to you and finding out for yourself what you feel has value.

When Sex Happens

Let's say that you end up engaging in conventional sex in spite of all guidance and vows; you either masturbate or make love with someone. As one of my teachers says, "Do it with awareness." (And remember contraceptive "training wheels" and safe sex guidance!)

If you can recover the nuance of sublimation, you might find yourselves drawing away from the conventional sexual behaviors that lead to orgasm and becoming quiet with each other. Tune in to your partner and yourself at the most subtle levels of sensation and allow your experiences to move in the direction of meditation.

Shift your bodily focus toward the base of your spine, heart, throat, or ajna chakra. Feel energy moving into your spine and within the chakras. You might find an energetic route different from the sexologist's path to the orgasmic point of no return. If you have proceeded blissfully toward the release and reflexes of orgasm, just enjoy it and take it all in. Later, you can make your way back to the passions of urdhvaretas. But at such times it is best to be with each other in the passions of desire.

Breaks can be an opportunity for unconditional self-acceptance and for accepting your partner, freed from perfectionist ideals. As Mike and Nancy discovered, couples brahmacharya yoga brings to the surface many of the same struggles that conventionally sexual couples face.

Mike and Nancy broke their vow of brahmacharya after seeing a movie—only R-rated at that. They were afraid to stop midway in their conventional lovemaking because they each felt that it was the other who "needed to be sexual." Neither wanted to "hurt" the other by frustrating or judging him or her. Yet they both hoped that the other would somehow draw away from sex, toward a tantric practice.

Their sexual exchange felt like it was part erotic mystery and love and part automatic habits. They fought about who was more disappointed by this slip, who really wanted to try brahmacharya more, and whose fault it was. Then they began apologizing as they felt how big erotic mystery really is, how, at times, it is even beyond our best intentions. They smiled and admitted liking having sex with each other. They decided that for a while at least, they would forego movies that might overcharge them in the conventional way.

Staying Loose, Playing, and Humor

> *I say unto you: one must still have chaos in oneself to be able to give birth to a dancing star.*
>
> NIETZSCHE,
> *THUS SPAKE ZARATHUSTRA*

Sex is one arena of life in which spontaneity comes out from hiding behind adult decorum and we let our hair down, for reasonless, spontaneous play is an extension of the child's innocent erotic life. With all the preparatory rituals, the structuring of position, breath, concentration, focus upon urdhvaretas and subtlety, how can we ever just "be" with each other? Indeed, a certain "transgressive" aspect of tantra is well known whereby the exhilarations of "breaking out" were explored in India, yet in ritualistically structured, brahmacharya-respecting and temporary ways.*

Playful contact, affection, comforting each other, and even massage are all forms of nonsexual touch. To find our answer to questions such as, "What about this kind of play? Or this kind of touch?" the judging or cynical mind, our own or that of others, must wait outside. "What is essential is often invisible to the eye," saith our foxy master. Ultimately, a trusting innocence will need to prevail.

Without needing to obsessively split hairs, we can discern the difference between playing lightheartedly in one's brahmacharya and toying with it. There will be a quiet or, at times, more obvious difference between affectionately teasing your partner and "getting at" him. In different contexts the same comment can be funny or not funny at all. Eros is always a matter of innuendo, and playful eros can become quite rough and in need of a little lightening up. Perhaps a simple apology and forgiveness will reveal the more freeing kind of play in no time. Remember to leave some nonexacting room for the dancing chaos.

Also, be aware of the tendency toward "preciousness." There is no reason to stop being earthy, juicy, and ordinary just because you are on the urdhvaretic way. Anyway, the throbs of prana and kundalini will change all *that*!

Support for Celibate Traditions in Modern Times

Except for those living on Mount Athos or elsewhere cloistered, modern monastics and celibate clergy are subjected to all manner of modern stimulations that can place great stress on their vows. Such simple and nonsectarian practices as alternate nostril breathing or yoni mudra (see page 212) can prove helpful in gathering one's energies.

---

*For more on this, see Wedemeyer, *Making Sense of Tantric Buddhism.*

Scientia Sexualis Desire and
Ars Erotica Sublimation Reconciled

Relating to a much larger social world that is pursuing the ways of sex-desire presents the tantric brahmacharyin with the danger of becoming judgmental of others. Why live this way if it isn't "superior" to "regular world sex?" one might ask. A tempting question, with a potentially heavy price to be paid if one tries to answer it, particularly while in a competitive mood.

Pursuing tantric brahmacharya while derogating sex-desire diminishes one's innocence. Such has been called "spiritual materialism": using meditative and other practices to feel superior to others. What good is any form of spiritual practice if it contributes to alienation or a condescending elitism? Any form of erotic mystery will always shrink from those who judge or shame it. Thus, the entire scientia sexualis must be objectively appreciated for what it is and is not.

You also cannot expect all the folks living in the scientia sexualis world around you to understand your ars erotica brahmacharya. Some living within the cynical certainties will choose to be suspicious of your claims of celibacy or will cringe that you are self-repressing, since they think they would never want to do what you are doing. Then there might be others involved in certain monastic paths who will question whether your tantric brahmacharya is pure enough. Make plenty of room in your heart for people to "not understand," as well as room for those who are curious, and even inspired to explore brahmacharya themselves.

Gradual Brahmacharya

To make the path to sublimative passion more accessible to a greater number of people who might otherwise remain unattracted to its mysteries, I offer a "gradual brahmacharya," a two-step approach to its precincts.

In the first step, all manner of conventional sexual activity can be explored, but the partners (or the individual) try to delete the endpoint known as genital orgasm from the exploration. A sort of endlessness can emerge, since this phase does not exhaust the partners in orgasm. Lovemaking can last many hours, with periods of meditation, breathing practices, and stretching included. If orgasm should occur, simply let go of what it might "mean." As stated throughout this book, the mood of worship is what shifts this coitus reservatus transitional stage from scientia sexualis to the endless ars erotica terra firma. But in all cases avoid the allure of cynicism and guilt. Merely proceed in continuing with your ars erotica ways, helping yourself and your partner. Remember, a monthly orgasmic exchange still fits the yogic energetic ecology of brahmacharya.

Gradually, in the second phase, more and more of the yogic practices are added to the lovemaking until the greater amount of time is spent with the rituals and meditations of tantric practice. The transition might be hardly noticeable; you suddenly find yourselves within the glow of urdhvaretas seed maturation. If you start missing sex, try just missing it. Feel the longing until it spreads into suggestive innuendos, then evanescent subtleties, and then desireless passion. If desire returns, you might be able to miss the wonder of urdhvaretas. Miss this wonder, feel the longing for it. And so on.

PROFUNDITY
WITHIN SIMPLICITY

Through worship you enter the retas mystery and manifest your deepest potentials. Growing ever deeper and wider into the felt meanings of *worship* is to mature the entheogenic rasas, the spinal puberties of perineum, heart, and mindspace. That is why I recommend that you worship daily, hourly, every second, in unrelenting gratitude and with complimentary words and actions, great and small, in asanas and kirtan or silent meditations, and so profoundly, with such longings of your soul, that you never want your worship to end, but to always blossom into more and endlessly more.

As my guru sang tearfully in the kavi-bhakti tradition regarding his own decades of yogic longings and transformation toward embodying the same maturity as Shiva-Shakti, the Lord of Yoga:

> I would like to become your feet when you walk . . . your eyes when you look . . . your tongue when you eat . . . your ears when you hear . . . your hands when you grasp something . . . your skin when you touch something . . . your nose when you smell a fragrance . . . [indeed,] to become a flower for your delicate touch. I would like to become a thin stream of the nectar of immortality. I would like to become a song in your throat, Shiva . . . to dance in beautiful clothes to make your eyes content. Oh Merciful One, I wish I could become your body, for you are my soul, my spirit and my consciousness . . . that is all I ask of you, that is all I ask of you.[4]

As all these images inspire you, you might find yourself getting up at 4 a.m. for hours of solo or partnered yoga practice and relational worship before work or child care or elder care begins. Those of you with others in your care can see them as retas-blossoming beings who break your heart open, over and over again with all they need and all they give to you. You can tell your friends, neighbors, work colleagues, clients, even your competitors, opposing counsel, "enemies" your most empathic or loving feelings, as each situation allows, however slim, over and over, in myriad ways. Become Shiva-Shakti; why not aim high?*

Thus, you will feel the profundity of retas mysteries within the daily simplicities of life, over and over again. You will also begin to see how the pain of interpersonal strife and even the tragedies of war can only emerge whenever this simplicity of "holding together as one whole family" is lost. May our appreciation and admiration of our close ones, for everyone, never cease, our empathies for their challenges ever deepen, and our worship grow wildly afire and with forgiveness for self and others wherever needed!

---

*For more on "aiming high," see Salzberg and Thurman, *Love Your Enemies: How to Break the Anger Habit & Be a Whole Lot Happier.*

Within the more intimate ars erotica realm, perhaps you and your partner will awaken the physical irresistibility between the two of you that goes on and on, always touching, smiling, always enjoying. Yoga practices are a part of it all, just as all our life is yoga, a manifestation of being conceived and born from profound retas energies combined in moments of gendered union, and bursting into this "other world" of ars erotica liberations and lifelong maturations. And perhaps the embodied heaven realm of Sringara Rasa will open during the spinal puberty and the entheogenic rasas will flow between you, as described in chapter 12, and interspersed throughout this book. Perhaps the asanas themselves will become spontaneous tumescences of lilting fingers and arching spines, as described in chapter 11. Perhaps in the decades ahead, the whole world will open up this ars erotica way, leaving "the austere monarchy of sex" and its "brave new world" far behind.

11
Hatha Yoga as Ars Erotica

Hatha yoga practices have been available in our culture for some time now, primarily as a form of gentle exercise or perhaps as physical disciplines that purify and prepare the body for meditation. To consider them as romantic-erotic practices is perhaps a semantical stretch, but only if we are bound up in the conventional understandings of eros. It is possible to animate our yogic practices, solitary or partnered, with the energy of bhakti-devotion and urdhvaretas-developmental passion. Yet yoga is rarely taught within this context. We usually learn poses as stretching exercises to hold and perfect, rather than as a repertoire of intimate and passionate gestures of love and self-expression that inherently perfect themselves as we incarnate ourselves more fully, "gestationally," with each asana and in between each asana.

I particularly encourage beginners to take a formal class. Although the ars erotica aspect would likely remain unexplored, the class will help bring the asanas to life and encourage your practice. I also recommend the following books: *Revealing the Secret* by Swami Kripalvananda, the *Ashtanga Yoga Primer* by Baba Hari Dass, and *Devatma Shakti* by Swami Vishnu Tirtha. People with special health conditions should consult a physician regarding specific practices and can refer to the

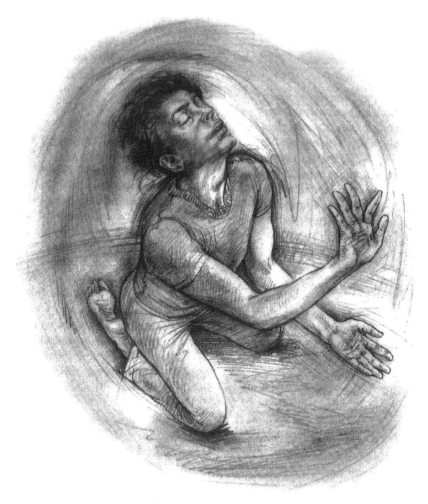

Yoga practice as ars erotica

above texts and B. K. S. Iyengar's *Light on Yoga* for contraindications for these and many other yoga practices.

BANDHAS AND MUDRAS

Bandhas (locks) are muscle contractions or, rather, tumescences that seal off specific areas of the body, thus enabling energies to go more deeply into our organs and subtle bodies. Watch for the subtle blissful feelings generated by any of the bandhas and discover other subtle internal contractions that further awaken such ars erotica arousals. Bandhas are performed in seated postures or as directed. In the descriptions of the practices, I make reference to specific breathing instructions in a shorthand manner. "KI" indicates *kumbhaka inhalation,* that is, briefly holding the breath "in" after inhaling, while "KO" indicates *kumbhaka exhalation,* briefly holding the breath "out" after exhaling.

 ### MULA BANDHA

1. Contract and lift inward the anal sphincter on an inhalation.
2. Hold (KI) for as long as comfortable, and release on the exhalation. This seals in the abdominal energy known as *apana pran* and conducts it upward toward manipura chakra, the site of transmutation; it is similar to Kegel exercises.

 ### JALANDHARA BANDHA

1. Press the chin into the hollow at the collarbone on an inhalation and hold (KI) or tumesce as long as comfortable to seal energy within the thorax and to preserve a subtle revitalizing nectar that flows through subtleties within the brachial vascular and neural plexuses down from the sahasrara.
2. Release chin-pressing during exhalation.

 ### UDDIYANA BANDHA

1. Exhale completely, draw the stomach muscles inward, and hold as long as is comfortable (KO).
2. Then slowly release the tumescent stomach muscles and the "upward flying" (*uddiyana*) breath.

 ### MAHA MUDRA

This practice employs all the above bandhas.

1. Sit with the right leg out straight and the left leg bent so that the sole touches the inner right thigh and the left heel presses the androgenous perineum.

2. Stretch the arms up, then lower arms forward to clasp the right toe with the thumbs and index fingers of both hands. Maintain concentration on ajna chakra.

3. Begin mula bandha during the inhalation, and hold the breath (KI) with jalandhara and uddiyana bandhas.

4. After exhalation, release mula, jalandhara, and uddiyana bandhas, then reapply uddiyana bandha, holding (KO) as long as is comfortable.

5. Then inhale, release your hands, and repeat, reversing leg positions. Begin with two rounds and increase to ten. Feel all the inner marriages celebrating their unions. Enter ars erotica secrecies of all secrecies: we are uroboric and reconceive ourselves!

 ### NABHAN MUDRA

Curl the tongue back so the tumescent tip touches the "little gateway" taluka point in the soft palate; this can be maintained along with many asanas and the bandhas to preserve subtle nectars and awaken the higher chakras. Taste Shiva-Shakti union as truth of the macrocosmic universe and your body-mind as the microcosm.

Pranayama

These breathing practices should be done sitting upright, cross-legged, or in a chair, with proper ventilation and preferably on an empty stomach. *Pranayama* is usually translated as "control (*yama*) of the breath (*prana*)," but yama is felt as a "savoring" of prana, thus "breath-savoring" is the more bhakti-based rendering.

 ### KAPALA-BHATI

In kapala-bhati the sacred prana of the head (udan pran) is "shined"; that is, made to glow its radiant vibrancies" (literally kapal is "skull" and bhati is "shine"). Use the in-drawn abdominal muscles to pump air out of the lungs forcefully, and passively release the abdomen to draw air in.

NADI SHODHANA SAHITA KUMBHAKA

This is an alternate nostril breath and is the single most important practice for brahmacharya. Use the right thumb to open and close the right nostril and the right ring finger and little finger to open and close the left. Maintain a ratio of 1:4:2 for the duration of each inhalation, hold (KI), and exhalation, beginning with 4 seconds to inhale, 16 seconds to hold, and 8 seconds to exhale.

1. Begin inhaling left, with the right nostril closed by the thumb, hold the breath, applying the mula bandha and jalandhara bandha while holding the breath in.
2. Then exhale through the right, closing the left nostril, and relax the locks when the breath is empty, for one second.
3. Then inhale through the right nostril and hold the breath while applying the locks. Then exhale left, and so on. A twenty-minute session is usually sufficient to balance various polarities and to stimulate the central nadis in and around the spine.

This pranayama balances energies that might have been excited through more vigorous practices. As ars erotica, nadi shodhana is a dialogue between the polarities of our being: left-right, yin-yang, female-male, moon-sun, *ida-pingala*. The inner marriage ceremony of sun and moon is hidden in the microcosm of the left and right bilaterality of your body and the androgyny of your perineum and hypothalamus.

ASANAS

All asanas will further the sublimative process. Choose the ones your particular body needs. Those that follow are especially helpful in brahmacharya. Center yourself with a few slow breaths, and move slowly to your capacity, wherever that may be. (Perhaps the asanas will emerge as ars erotica tumescences, arising of their own accord, sahaja.)

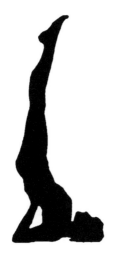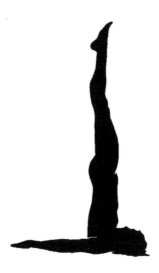

 ## VIPARITA KARANI MUDRA (REVERSE POSE TUMESCENCE)

1. Lie on your back. While inhaling, raise your legs to a vertical position and, with your elbows on the floor, support your hips with your hands and hold as long as is comfortable, breathing normally. (See left figure.)
2. Lower slowly on exhalation. In the shoulder stand (sarvanga-asana) continue raising your upper back off the floor and use your hands to support your raised back, balanced comfortably on your shoulders. (See right figure.) Hold.
3. Lower your back slowly, using your hands as a brace.

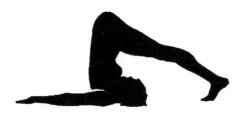

 ## HALA-ASANA (PLOW POSE TUMESCENCE)

1. From the reverse pose, exhale slowly and lower your legs down over your head. Keep your knees straight, and straighten your arms flat onto the floor, parallel with your body.

2. Continue lowering your legs until your toes touch the floor. Hold this position and breathe slowly.

3. Reverse the movement to come out of the pose.

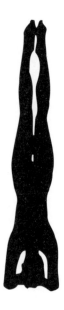

 SHIRSA-ASANA (HEADSTAND TUMESCENCE)

Unless you are already competent in this especially useful pose, I strongly recommend learning it with an instructor.

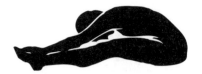

 PASCHIMOTTANA-ASANA (SEATED HEAD-TO-KNEE, BACK-STRETCHING POSE TUMESCENCE)

This one is also known as brahmacharya-*asana*.

1. Sitting on the floor with your legs straight out, inhale while raising your arms up; stretch and hold.

2. Then exhale while reaching out and forward, lowering your torso and head

to your legs, clasp your big toes with your index finger and thumb. Perform uddiyana bandha and hold the pose.

3. Inhale while raising and stretching up, then lower your arms as you exhale.

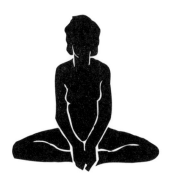

 ### BHADRA-ASANA (NOBILITY POSE TUMESCENCE)

1. Sitting upright, press the soles of your feet together, and hold your feet with your hands, drawing them close to your body.

2. Inhale and press your knees toward the floor, and hold.

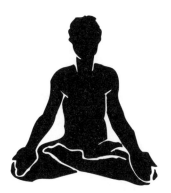

 ### PADMA-ASANA (LOTUS POSE TUMESCENCE)

1. Sit on the floor with your legs crossed. Lift your left foot onto your right thigh, placing it as near to your hip as possible without straining; lift your right foot onto your left thigh. Women should reverse the leg position, placing the left foot on top.

2. Rest your hands on your knees, keeping your back straight.

SIDDHA-ASANA (ADEPT POSE TUMESCENCE)

1. Women: Bend your left leg so that your left heel presses your perineum; then bend your right leg, placing your right foot on top of the left foot, pressing your pubic bone.
2. Men: Follow the instructions for women, but reverse left and right leg positions.

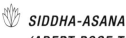 ### *YOGA MUDRA (GESTURE OF UNION TUMESCENCE)*

1. Kneeling or in lotus pose, inhale as your arms float behind your back; clasp your hands and raise your arms behind you from the shoulders, stretching.
2. Exhale and lower your torso and head to the floor in front of you (KO).
3. Rest, then inhale, raising your torso fully, and release your arms.

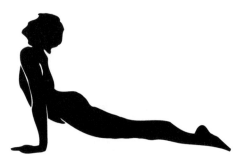

 ### *SARA HASTA BHUJANGA-ASANA (KING COBRA TUMESCENCE)*

1. Lying flat on your stomach in the push-up position, inhale, raising first only your head, then your shoulders.
2. Then, pressing your hands into the floor, raise your torso, arching up and back as comfortably as possible, while keeping your pelvis pressed into the floor.
3. Stretch your eyes by looking up, and hold, and exhale while slowly lowering. In the cobra (bhujanga-asana), raise your torso three-quarters of the way up.

Beginner to Intermediate
Series of Asanas

The basic twenty willful postures, as well as the postures for the more experienced, catalogued in the chart on the following pages, were given to me through the grace and good wishes of yogis in the lineage of Swami Kripalvananda. Both series systematically strengthen the bodily domains of each chakra by employing specific pranayama instructions and concentrations for each asana.

Each asana should be practiced two to five times or held for one to five minutes, as indicated on the chart. In repeated asanas, inhale while completing the expansive movement and hold after inhaling (KI). Then exhale on lowering movements for each posture and hold the breath out (KO).

Where KI-KO is noted for asanas that are held for one to five minutes, breathe in the completed pose, holding the breath at both the fully inhaled and fully exhaled points of each breath; "normal breath" during a held asana means just that. Begin coming out of the asana on an inhalation, as you move into the next with as few transitional movements or breaths as possible.

During the first six months, the basic twenty postures or series for the more experienced should be practiced without the chakra concentrations. Thereafter, attention should be paid to the concentration points and to any spontaneously arising bandhas or pranayamas. After approximately one year of daily or twice daily practice, the series can be done in an unbroken sequence, using only one breath during the transition from one posture to the next. If the lotus posture is uncomfortable, you may adapt a simple cross-legged position where indicated.

BASIC TWENTY POSTURES

Asana	Chakra	Duration	Kumbhaka
yoga mudra in lotus	muladhara	2–5x	KI, KO
back-stretching (*pashchimottana-asana*)	muladhara	2–5x	KI, KO
spinal twist (*ardha-matsyendra-asana*)	svadhisthana	1–5 min each side	normal breath
mountain pose (*buddha-padma-asana*)	svadhisthana	2–5x	KO
lotus-swing (*lola-asana*)	manipura	2–5x	KI
lotus-balance chin lock (*dola-asana*)	manipura	1–5 min	KI, KO
lotus lying on back (*ardha-supta-padma-asana*)	manipura	1–5 min	KI, KO
fish (*matsyana-asana*)	anahata	1–5 min	KI, KO
reverse pose, lotus (*viparita karani-padma-asana*)	anahata	1–5 min	normal breath
plow (*hala-asana*)	vishuddha	1–5 min	normal breath
knee-ear (*karani pida-asana*)	vishuddha	1–5 min	normal breath
shoulder stand (*sarvanga-asana*)	vishuddha	1–5 min	normal breath
reverse, legs inclined posterior (*viparita karani*)	vishuddha	1–5 min	KI, KO
gas release pose (*mukta pavana-asana*)	vishuddha	1–5 min	KI
bridge (*setu-asana*)	ajna	2–5x	KI
cobra, legs apart toes curled under (*bhujanga-asana*)	ajna	2–5x	KI
locust (*salabha-asana*)	ajna	2–5x	KI
bow (*dhanura-asana*)	ajna	2–5x	KI, KO
headstand (*sirsa-asana*)	sahasrara	1–5 min	normal breath
relaxation (*sava-asana*)	vishuddha	1–5 min	normal breath

FOR THE MORE EXPERIENCED

Asana	Chakra	Duration	Kumbhaka
head-to-knee, standing (pada hasta-asana)	manipura	2–5x	KO
back-stretching (pashchimottana-asana)	manipura	2–5x	KI, KO
spinal twist left, right (ardha matsyendra-asana)	manipura	1–3 min each side	normal breath
yoga mudra in lotus (yoga mudra)	muladhara	2–5x	KI, KO
lotus balance chin lock (dola-asana)	manipura	1–5 min	KI, KO
fish in lotus (padma matsya-asana)	anahata	5x	KI
reverse pose, lotus (viparita karani padma-asana)	vishuddha	5x	KI, KO
fold down in lotus (chirsprishta-asana)	vishuddha	5x	normal breath
knee-ear (karani pida-asana)	vishuddha	1–5 min	normal breath
plow (hala-asana)	ajna	1–5 min	normal breath
shoulder stand (sarvanga-asana)	ajna	2–5 min	KI, KO
reverse pose (viparita karani mudra)	vishuddha	1–3 min	KI, KO
gas-release pose (mukta pavana-asana)	manipura	5x	KI
navel-gaze pose, lying on back (nabhidara shana-asana)	manipura	1–3 min	KI
relaxation pose (sava-asana)	vishuddha	1 min	normal breath
king cobra, legs apart, toes curled under (sara hasta bhujanga-asana)	manipura	5x	KI, KO
cobra, legs apart, toes curled under (bhujanga-asana)	ajna	5x	KI, KO
locust (salabha-asana)	manipura	5x	KI, KO
bow (dhanura-asana)	manipura	5x	KI, KO
headstand (sirsa-asana)	sahasrara	1–5 min	normal breath
relaxation pose (sava-asana)	vishuddha	1 min	normal breath

I generally suggest one hour of daily practice. Two hours per day is a minimum if you would like to see the effects that are possible if yoga becomes a central factor in your life. Of course, there are lesser known tips, like doing one round of alternate nostril breathing at red lights or during commercials (or even during regular TV for the more ascetic types), doing inner mantra meditation while waiting in lines, and so forth. Meditative awareness can also be practiced during the day by tuning in to the subtleties of the colors, sounds, interpersonal communications, and so forth of the external world.

The more formal daily practices should also be done—should, the most maligned guidepost of modern times. Can we be disciplined and regular without getting compulsive? Can we employ techniques yet stay open to the mercurial and serendipitous mystery?

THE NOT-ENOUGH-TIME ROUTINE

Practice daily is the golden rule of yoga. So to keep things rolling when you are in a pinch, here is a suggested fifteen-minute routine.

1. Sit down and forget the rush. Do one hundred rounds of kapala-bhati in sets of ten or more, according to your comfort, holding the breath out for a few seconds after each set, with the mula and jalandhara bandhas, then holding the last breath in for a longer time, with the locks.
2. Then do two different asanas, holding each posture for about three minutes, with a rest in between.
3. For the rest of the time, five to eight minutes, do very relaxed, nadi shodhana sahita kumbhaka pranayama.

An Advanced Series of Practices

Following is a set of advanced pranayama and purification practices that balance the sub-pranas and stimulate the nadis and chakras in a close sequence in preparation for meditation. These practices, as taught by Baba Hari Dass, will be more useful for those with at least one year of yoga experience.

GHARSHANA PRANAYAMA

1. Inhale nasally from the chest and exhale by drawing the stomach muscles in, controlling the breath with the glottis (*ujjayi* breath), which produces a soothing, hissing-sighing sound in the throat.
2. Do ten breaths, then do ten rounds of alternate nostril breathing without retention (kumbhaka).
3. Repeat this sequence.
4. Then proceed to the next exercise.

CHATUR BHUJA PRANAYAMA

1. Do ten rounds of alternate nostril breathing, of equal duration on inhaling and exhaling and holding out the breath (KO) each time for the count of ten; that is, 10:10:10.
2. Then proceed to the next exercise.

MAHA MUDRA, AGNISARA DHAUTI, MAHA VEDHA MUDRA

This is an excellent series for urdhvaretas.

1. Do maha mudra to the right outstretched leg, holding inhalation (KI).
2. Then move to the lotus, exhaling, and hold the breath out (KO) for one breath while pumping the stomach muscles in and out repeatedly. This is *agnisara dhauti.*
3. Then inhale in lotus, and use your hands against the floor on each side of you to raise your body off the floor, holding the inhalation (KI), and apply mula bandha and jalandhara bandha to your limit, and lower, exhaling. This is *maha vedha mudra.*
4. Repeat maha mudra to the left leg, and go through the same sequence.
5. Repeat the whole sequence two to five times, ending with maha mudra to the right leg.
6. Then proceed to the next exercise.

ASVINI MUDRA

1. In siddha asana contract and relax the anal sphincter, as in mula bandha, fifty times on an in-held breath (KI).
2. Then proceed to the next exercise.

 ## YONI MUDRA

1. Using your thumbs, index fingers, middle, ring, and little fingers to close your ears, eyelids, nostrils, and upper and lower lips, take in a slow full breath and hold, pressing very gently against the eyelids on the lower edge of the bony socket (not on the cornea) to release eye tension in a flourish of colors and patterns. Watch them in meditative wonder. This completes the yoni mudra.
2. Then on the next inhalation proceed to the next exercise.

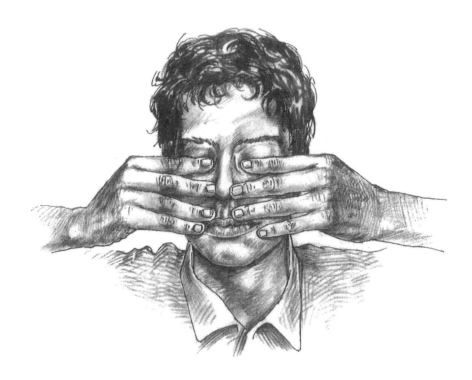

Yoni mudra

CHAKRA ACTIVATION

1. Begin concentrating on a point outside your body below the base of your spine, and internally say the mantra "humg" (ending with a nasal "mg") while bringing your attention to muladhara chakra; enter into the center of the chakra with the mantra "hamg" (ending with a nasal "mg") and feel the blossoming of the chakra open with the mantra "sahhh."
2. Repeat the combination of mantras and concentration exercises at each chakra, concluding with ajna chakra.
3. Then return to muladhara chakra to repeat the whole sequence.

BHASTRIKA

1. Perform a slow, full, deep inhalation with the silent mantra of "swaaa" and an exhalation with the silent "haaa." Do this for ten rounds.
2. Then proceed to the next exercise.

MEDITATION FOR ALL

1. Meditation on ajna chakra balances all other chakras by attuning them to the nondual poise of this center. Svadhisthana, often called the "sexual center" by scientia-immersed yogis, matures ars erotically and comes more into balance in this attunement. Hold the nabhan mudra and occasionally the mula bandha. This is the esoteric anatomical basis for why women place "bindi dots" on their midbrow points and yogis smear their foreheads with sandalwood pastes and ash to symbolize retas has been fully activated and burned all the way down to ashes.
2. Meditate upon the deity as the essence of mother, father, spouse, sister, brother, daughter, son, friend, lover, foe, teacher, student.
3. Meditate upon the serene radiance of the moon as a source of coolly reflected sunlight; the essence of the unexplored forest; the blue of a cloudless sky; the flowing invisibility of crystal water of an unwavering flame; the milky, golden richness of a flowing nectar; the first rays of a sunrise and last rays of a sunset; the subtle movements of a sleeping animal or infant; the cosmic rhythms beyond choices and desires.

CHAIR AND BED
YOGA

Age and physical condition are not limitations to the full blossoming of the seed force, a blossoming that is always lifelong, inclusive of even our last moments. Following are some practices that can be tried when more strenuous activity is not possible.

 ## *LEG LIFTS*

1. Raise your leg slowly on the inhalation, hold with locks, and lower on the exhalation.
2. Raise your legs a few inches or more but never strain yourself. If needed, hold the ends of a six-foot-long cloth, stretched under your knees, and raise and lower your legs with the cloth. Concentrate on manipura.

 ## *SHOULDER, NECK, WRIST, ANKLE, AND HIP ROTATIONS*

1. Rotate shoulder, neck, wrist, ankle, and hips slowly in synchrony with breathing.
2. Reverse the direction of rotation.

 ## *EYE ROTATION AND ROLLING*

1. Rotate your eyes and roll them up and down while visualizing the sublimative flow of energies throughout the body.

 ## *MOVING WITH THE BREATH*

1. Squeeze and relax fists and feet, with the in and out breaths.
2. Undulate the spine with the breath, and concentrate on various chakras.

For those unable to move physically, meditation upon the images of asanas, perhaps while viewing a video course, can induce some of the effects of performing the asanas within the causal, mental, vital, and physical bodies.

FAMILY PRACTICE
IDEAS

- Along with grace before meals, try three rounds of rhythmic or alternate nostril breathing.
- Using a children's yoga book as a guide, practice asanas together, with favorite music in the background.
- Have the younger members of the family teach the older ones a new stretch or other practice.
- See what prenatal yoga books (or classes) have to offer. Practice of asvini mudra, bhadra asana, and nadi shodhana are generally helpful to prepare for labor and delivery. This goes for fathers as well as mothers.

PARTNERED
PRACTICES

Enjoy the close nonverbal rapport of sensing physical limitations while providing gentle support to maintain and deepen any stretch. Breathe and even sigh with each other, and sense the release of tensions during the holding of any position. In balance poses use the breath to lighten yourselves, and focus your gaze on a stable point several yards away from you. Conclude a series of asanas by resting a comfortable degree of your full chest weight on the back of your partner, who is in child-pose (kneeling with the head resting face down on the floor and arms extending alongside the legs with the palms facing up). Please note that the partnered practices in this section are contemporary adaptations of yogic and other stretching practices.

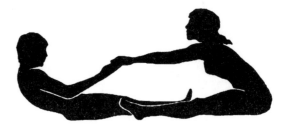

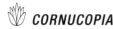 **CORNUCOPIA**

1. Sit on the floor facing your partner with your legs spread wide, holding your partner's legs apart with the edge of your feet on her knees or ankles; reach out and clasp hands to the wrists.
2. As one of you slowly leans backward, the other comes forward; slowly move this leaning into a rotating movement, from the torso. Circle to the left and to the right. Breathe deeply, slowly, and rhythmically, concentrating on manipura when you are leaning back and on anahata when you are upright. Make the sound "mmmm" when leaning back and "aaahhhhh" when coming upright.

You might be able to feel a radiant field of pulsation around each other's genitals. You can discern how urdhvaretic passion permeates this radiance with a natural rapport of spontaneous blending, while sex-desire passion will make you feel you are lacking something and need to get closer in order to end the longing. It might feel like a rhythm of its own, hidden within your first sensings of the radiance around each other's genitals and svadhisthana chakra areas.

Allow this union to keep spreading throughout your bodies and into the retas, subtle and profound. This will add a gracefulness to your rowing movements and may make them utterly effortless and mysteriously erotic, yet without desire. You might be able to distinguish the procreative passion that pulses within your bodies in synchrony with ovulation-menstrual, lunar, and spermatogenic cycles.

These shared feelings and stretches can permeate chronic tension of back muscles, sometimes called sexual tension, and cause a pleasant release. Just give in to the stretch and gradually let go of the back pain and rigidity. The ars erotica passion between the two of you will give you a key to this release. Womb, ovaries, and testicles also benefit from the relaxed stretching and movements.

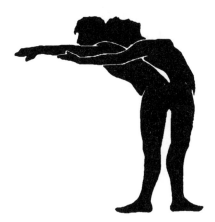

 HEARTS AND BACKS

1. Stand back to back with your partner; reach your arms up and have your partner reach up and clasp you at the elbows or wrists, whichever is easier.

2. Before lifting your partner completely onto your back, test his weight to ensure your capacity to hold and balance him in the full position. Then bend forward very slowly on an exhalation, slightly lifting your partner onto your back and onto his toes, stretching open his chest.

3. The underneath person: hold the exhalation out (KO) and perform (or "tumesce") stomach lifts, uddiyana bandha. The raised person will feel an opening of his chest around the heart. Sigh with any sensations of stretching in this area, and feel the vibrations of your sighing ripple through your heart area. The sighing can become more and more expressive of feelings from your heart as they spread into your throat and down into your belly. Your partner will feel the vibrations of any sighing and might join in.

4. Hold in this stretch, concentrating on anahata and feeling the connection of hearts, from back to back. You can also stretch your held arms slightly open to the sides, and then back toward the center, with the breath. Breathe with the sound "llllllllllmmmmmmmmmm," from time to time, relaxing your throats and voices. Also, be aware of the contact points at the buttocks and back of the head.

5. After one to five minutes, exchange positions by rolling slowly upright.

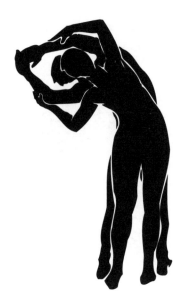

 ### CRESCENT MOON

1. Begin the same as in Hearts and Backs, but stretch slowly and laterally to the left, then to the right, from the torso, in synchrony with the breath. Feel contact points at coccyx, back of heart area, and heads. Converse silently with energy and feeling through these points.

2. Rock slowly and laterally from left to right to left, and become increasingly aware of manipura. Apply the anal lock (mula bandha) at each extreme of the stretch, and release the lock as you come to center.

3. The stretch is in the sides; the activation point of movement is at the navel. Find a rhythm to your lateral, swaying movement; as you do so, feel a balancing of yin and yang, female and male, left and right, moon and sun, objects and space. With each sweep, feel ars erotica passion swelling until your movements have become childlike and playful.

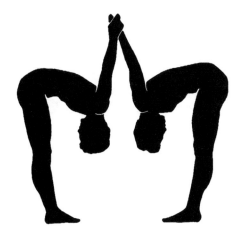

 ## *DUAL YOGA MUDRA, STANDING*

1. Stand facing each other, feet shoulder-width apart, at such a distance that when you bend forward at the waist toward each other, your heads nearly touch. While erect, inhale very slowly as you float (tumesce) your hands behind your own backs; clasp your hands behind you, concentrate on muladhara, and slowly bend forward on the exhalation, bringing your head down toward your knees.

2. Then reach your hands up and across to grasp each other at the wrists or forearms, and hold in this position, gently stretching down with your head and neck, and gently pulling at each other's wrists or arms. Feel the presence of your partner's head near your own and the field of space that you share surrounding your heads. Feel the sensations of energy flowing in your spine and perhaps even in your partner's spine. Feel the blood flowing into your head, and scan your legs and feet.

3. You can experiment with holding your breaths out (KO) and applying the three locks (bandhas), sensing any responses in muladhara. Feel the vibrations of energy at those times radiating up each other's arms as you hold your breath out.

4. Come up slowly, when you want to, on an inhalation, first releasing your partner's wrists, and then exhale as you approach standing position, while your arms float around to your sides.

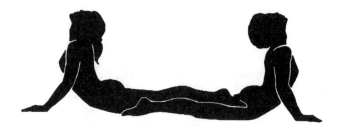

 ## TWIN COBRAS

1. Together, you each do the cobra while facing opposite directions and away from each other, with one person's legs outside of the other's and resting on top of the inside partner's legs to hold them down.

2. Raise your torsos up slowly, together, on an inhalation, and concentrate on svadhisthana on the way up, pressing your pelvises into the floor. You will feel your genitals, womb, or ovaries pressing down into the earth at this time. Feel the earth's energy and massive security holding the two of you in a rapport of giving and receiving through your pelvises.

3. When you have raised your torsos and are each supporting your weight with your arms in the full cobra, move your concentration to ajna. Forget your partner completely. Just concentrate on ajna, with your eyes rolled up, open or closed. Hold and hold (KI).

4. Then lower on an exhalation. Repeat three to ten times, alternating your leg position with that of your partner.

5. You can also raise (tumesce) in the twisting cobra, by shifting your head and shoulders left, snakelike, then right, then left, all the way up into the completed cobra pose.

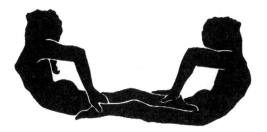

 TWIN BOATS

1. This is similar to the twin cobras, but instead of supporting yourself on your hands, reach your hands behind you to the top of your partner's heels. As you come up on the inhalation (KI), hold onto each other's heels and pull slightly.

2. You can each bend your legs slightly at the knee to draw your partner up a little more, if the extra stretch is needed. You can even start closer together; then bending the knees to give additional stretching to the arms and legs will be easier. Concentration is on manipura.

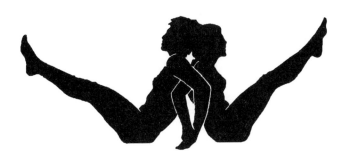

 URDHVARETAS "V"

1. Sit on the floor back to back with your legs together and straight out. Hook your arms at the elbow, both of you pressing your hands to the floor. Lean into each other at the head and shoulders, press your palms firmly against the floor, and raise up your legs on a slow inhalation, so you are in a "V" pose. (Raising your legs just a few inches is sufficient in the beginning.)

2. Hold, and do thirty rounds of kapala-bhati breath, then hold the last inhalation

(KI) and apply the three locks (bandhas). Bring the energy to manipura, and feel the glowing bliss.

3. Lower on the exhalation, and repeat three to twenty times.

This can be done with pillow supports under your raised legs in order to hold the pose longer. If using pillows, raise and lower your legs briefly, bending at the knees if necessary. This is a strenuous practice that awakens ardor of ars erotica longings. Start slowly.

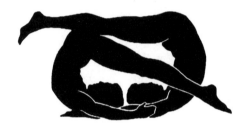

TWIN PLOWS

1. Lie straight out on your backs, head to head, and reach back to hook arms at the elbows. Raise up into the Reverse Pose (page 203), and feel the energy and blood supply lower into the abdomen, adrenal glands, kidneys, liver. Let the blood flow out of the legs.

2. Continue up to Shoulder Stand (page 203), touching at the ankles for balance, and concentrate on ajna. Then lower your legs back over your head and into the plow (page 203). One partner's legs come to rest on either side of the other's buttocks, and the other rests her legs on her partner's buttocks. Feel the harmony of this balance and the opening of the vertebrae.

3. Breathe and sigh in this pose, gently rocking each other, with micromotions. You can return to a shoulder stand and then lower into the plow again, reversing the position of your legs to give you each a leg stretch to the floor.

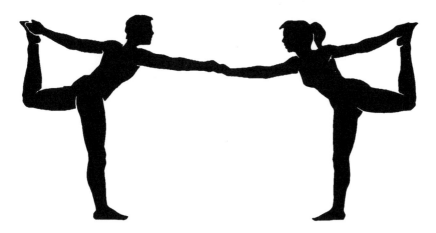

 TWIN DANCERS' POSE

1. Stand facing each other at a distance that allows your outstretched arms to meet in wrist grips. Hold this position, right hand to right hand.
2. Then lift your left leg behind you, bending the knee, and clasp it with your left hand. You will be balancing with each other to accomplish this. Drawing your leg up and up with your arm completes this most graceful ars erotica pose.
3. To help maintain your balance, fix your focus on a spot on the floor or wall until you come down, on an exhalation. Reverse and repeat.

You will have to adjust for differences in weight and size, but, theoretically, any two people can come into balance for increasingly longer periods of time once they discover how to work together. Children with adults find this a great practice. In fact, most of these ars erotica practices can be done with all members of the family, over the age of four, without discomfort.

Practice Space

I encourage you to allow the spontaneity of ars erotica passion to lead you into further improvisations. Erotic life suffers under constant regimentation. In fact, you may want to fashion a "foam playground" space to replace the thin and narrow mat you might be currently using. Modern yoga mats are too confining for spontaneously emerging asanas. Indeed, Hasidic davening; Sufi zikr; esoteric belly dancing;

Pentacostal or Holy Ghost gospel church services; African, Dionysian, and a host of other cultural esoteric trance-dance forms could all also be explored.

SAHAJA YOGA

> 50. *Though he performs all actions, he is not bound by them, as a lotus leaf in the water is not touched by it.*
> 51. *That is called action of the body in which reason takes no part and which does not originate as an idea springing in the mind.*
> 52. *To speak simply, yogis perform actions with their bodies, like the movements of children.*
>
> JNANESHVARI

In ars erotica sahaja yoga we discover that the postures, breathing practices, and meditations can become natural tumescences within urdhvaretas. The spirit or quality of passion that we bring to these practices is as significant as the practices themselves. How, then, to find this passion?

The purist approach consists of meditating in stillness until your body begins to move on its own, however long that might take, sometimes called "awaiting the beloved." This approach simulates how many yoga postures originated, with a spontaneity similar to stretching in bed while barely awake. Here the stillness of meditation allows prana, the vital energy of prana-maya kosha, to build to a certain pitch, and then, guided by its inner intelligence, prana moves the body exactly as it needs to be moved to release tensions and blocked emotions and embody longings and the many moods of aspiration and inspiration. We are assured of entrance into urdhvaretas passion through the immediacy of movement itself. The grace of each articulating finger-tilt, wrist-twist, leg-lift, neck-turn opens *nadis* (subtle channels) and stimulates the chakras. The yogic movements feel like acts of surrendered worship and each asana a bodily form of prayer. However, not everyone can arouse prana through meditation to such a degree that spontaneous, or sahaja, yoga results.

There are several ways the breath can be willfully managed in the beginning as an entrance to the more spontaneous movements. Perhaps the easiest way is to move very slowly into a series of asanas while breathing just as slowly as you are moving. Synchronizing breath, movement, and concentration engages prana, and at some point you will feel as if you are no longer willfully moving but are being moved by prana itself. As you penetrate mundane thinking by mentally merging with the nuances of bodily sensation, you will slip unobtrusively into a meditative state. In this way postures and variations unfold in the moment as a flow from one asana to another known in yoga as *vinyasa* (posture flow).

A third way to discover sublimative passion is through building up prana through vigorous yogic breathing such as kapala-bhati or bhastrika as described above. After completing a series of these energizing breaths, you will feel a strong charge of energy or a dominant emotion and can begin moving with these feelings into various asanas until the spontaneity of movement is triggered.

Sometimes the prolonged suspension of the breath (kumbhaka) or merely sighing very deeply with each exhalation can rouse this passion. Another way is to use specific exercises that systematically stimulate the five fields of pranas—head (*udana*), chest (*prana*), midtorso (*samana*), abdomen (*apana*), and circulatory (*vyana*)—and various nadis and chakras through a precise sequence of yoga practices as in the experienced routine given above.

Another way to arouse prana is by holding a posture in increasingly more accurate alignment. Here, perfecting an asana is like perfectly attuning an instrument to a certain key. When the pitch becomes perfect, strong vibrations of energy can be felt, and one asana follows another, according to our specific needs. Holding a posture beyond the first limits of discomfort can trigger yogic passion and spontaneous asanas and pranayamas, and even dance movements. We must give ourselves permission to move, even with the scantiest of internal guidance. Or the spontaneous asanas might just tumesce pervasively, as labor contractions arise when baby wants out, according to Kripalvananda:

During meditation one experiences that by taking away the mind's control over the body, various organs of the body begin to perform activities. One or both hands may begin to be lifted slowly; one or both legs are stretched without one's will; the body bends down without one's doing so; one begins to rock or tremble or sing or laugh without apparent cause . . . or start performing various *asanas, mudras,* and *pranayamas* without having learned them. One observes all these activities during meditation with wonder.[1]

Muktananda describes his experience this way:

"[My] legs suddenly moved into *padmasana* . . . and [my] tongue curled up into [my] inner nasal passage. . . . I tried to get up and run away, but I couldn't because my legs were locked in lotus pose."[2]

Other more subtle contractions of the abdominal muscles draw sexual energy to manipura, an important site of transmutation, and also can cause the intercostal muscles to flex with subtle pleasures, propelling energies farther into the nadis in the thorax. Various pumping motions in the throat, rib cage, sacrum, lumbar, and perineum, along with micromotion of the eyelids, nasal muscles, fingers, toes, head, and even the scalp, carry the urdhvaretas seed energies throughout the whole body. Again, it is the nuances that bring a depth of feeling and expression to each movement, revealing its pleasures and meanings.

Finally, it becomes clear that you are moving from one sahaja activity to another, expressing urdhvaretas passion in your own perfect way. Perhaps it will take the form of rotating the neck while drawing the breath in, then exhaling the humming sound of "hmmmm" in your throat, which vibrates into a smile as you release the breath and stretch forward on the floor into the cobra posture, then draw your legs up under you to sit cross-legged in stillness, followed by an elaborate series of finger and hand movements, in which moods change with every tilt of each finger, myriad variations, each unique to the moment. Thus some yoga texts claim that there are 840,000 yoga asanas.

Gradually we achieve a bodily openness and a rechanneling of erotic pleasures that transform our practiced sublimation into a natural brahmacharya. We feel more free of the tugs and pulls of scientia sexualis culture because we feel more fullness in ourselves, and we are more appreciative of what we are already receiving from others. *This* is the yoga of the millennia!

12
Sringara Rasa

Warning: Highly susceptible to scientia reductionism, these explorations can release cosmic bonding power too great to share with anyone except harmonious "till death do us part" ars erotically matured partners.

> *First slowly with kisses everywhere,*
> *the dripping ahead hours lost in time*
> *this way then that, passage-ways opening*
> *flooding unfurling wrists held down and*
> > *released*
> *this that um yes and yes*
> *and suddenly you on top at two a.m. there it is,*
> *the frenzy, the shameless unabashed selfish freedom of*
> > *it all comes out*
> *wild almost hideous the truth of yes wanting*
> > *mmmmmore,*
> *whispering head turned this way more, then that way*
> > *more,*
> *even after the third hour, more more and yes of course,*
> *the more you take the better it is,*
> *for here in this endless place, more is all there is.*

Devouring each other upward,
ascending the spinal tree of knowledge, of life—elan
    vital itself,
becomes the (secret) maturational pathway
for the evermore incarnating spirit—
all the way up from lingam and yoni
to the crown, the radiant jewel,
the conduit: a river of concentration
surging inward vibrating serpentine Kundalini-shakti

Source-turned surging through the violet-tinged
    perineum trikonam
("triangular city of fire, flashing forth like lightning
    bolts
and resembling molten gold" Goraksha Paddhati
    1.20)
and up the milky-white spinal cord
into the cranial heaven-realms of erogenous mind
vaginal-satiny brain flesh
seething sulci thousand-petaled orgasms
beyond the covered in shame garbled tales of Genesis
all the way up to drink the pineal soma-rasa
nectar of the gods alchemical elixir, heady froth

I recall the kisses, so deliberate
slowly focusing our lips upon one another
watching your lips like petals falling as if
they were fainting into themselves
into another place far far away—
Those lips, wanting more, awaiting more,
this way then that, tongue flicks here and there
then opening into the warm moist cathedral of joined
    mouths
licking slowly the inside your cheeks,
beneath your tongue

drinking each other delicately and then thirstily,
years, decades of thirst coming out.
Pausing, returning, looking hands grazing your
    breasts
as you leaning leaned further toward me
the tunnel of your deep neckline suddenly dropping
    down
opening that chasm, the darkness in the center,
your breasts revealed indirectly as you crawled toward
    me
closing the distance fully desiring whether you knew it
    or not
for me to see, look, take, please,
reach into me as I reach into you.

Then came the cumming of mouths pulsing profusely
    into each other
drinking madly mysterious and rare
liquid lilacs intoxicating delirious
madhu mead the honey-wine amrita nectar of the
    gods
saturating into each other's slaked thirst.

The more the drinking in, the thirstier we became
You drinking my drinking of your drinking of my
    drinking
getting to the last hidden dram
of floral sweetness lurking deep inside the funneled
    blossom
stamen pistils gold-pollen-flecked anthers,
xylem tubules and micro-tubules patiently conducting
the earthy-dew into itself and phloem nourishing back
    downward
into the roots, root-hairs, in dark twining intercourse
    with soil muck

feeling up the crystalline sand grains
nubile vibrating constantly hard wet and quivering
then back up xylem, the ruddy menstrual wine, ferric,
the sweat of us, saline licked and re-licked tenderly,
other nectars of you of me, I want them all forever.

SUGGESTIVE AMBIGUITIES OF TWILIGHT TEACHINGS REVEAL, CONCEAL, AND PROTECT THE INTIMUS

Sringara Rasa, "Ars Erotica Heaven Realm," points to a long-term state shared by a couple, a whole community, or even a whole "world and era" of urdhvaretically maturing and matured persons. References to Sringara Rasa are found in certain multilayered bhakti and tantric twilight teachings, where *twilight* refers to teachings half hidden in metaphors that puzzle scholars as to their "reality."* For example, are the depictions in Tibetan *tangka* (sacred paintings) of male-female Yab-Yum unions, surrounded by flames, with the partners' eyes ablaze in all-chakra love, meant to represent actual human couples, or do they represent deities only, or are they esoteric symbols pertaining to human-deity meditative spirit-unions, or (merely) inner marriage meditative states? Or are the famed Khajuraho Temple carvings of couples and groups engaged in ars erotica worship merely "sex education" for monks returning to worldly life, as noted at the website for Khajuraho tourism,

---

*For more on the ambiguities and hidden, nonverbal subtleties of twilight teachings, see *The Twilight Language* by Roderick S. Bucknell and Martin Stuart-Fox; and Roger Jackson's critical review of their book in *The Journal of the International Association of Buddhist Studies* 11, no. 2 (1988): 123–30. For broader discussions on twilight ambiguities, see the works on *différance,* as coined by the French philosopher Jacques Derrida via Sanskritist Saussure et al., that point to subtleties, secrecies, and mutabilities of oral, in-the-moment communication between people, such as a living exchange between a tantric guru and her student—essential, undeterminable, and interminable differences—that can easily be lost in their permanent inscription in written text or remain in *samdhyabhasa,* the controversial "twilight language" of wisely hidden tantric teachings. (See Derrida, *"Différance," Margins of Philosophy.*)

or is this a bowdlerized public relations spin that conceals ars erotica, whole-community mysteries once led by powerful tantric gurus under the guise of the inapplicable, tourist-directed term, "*sex* education"?*

Or more wisely, if not cunningly, have the ancients resorted to half-revealed, half-concealed twilight conveyance of these Sringara and pariyanga teachings to protect them from age-old-to-present snickering misperceptions, narrow-minded pruderies, and merely lascivious or immature corruptions, while also beneficently leaving traces behind intelligible only to those whose urdhvaretic maturity can make sense of them, with tears of awe and felt-confirmation flowing?† Here is an example from the *Thirumandiram* of Siddhar Thirumoolar (rendered ars erotically by me) so you can see for yourself.

825. *Pleasure of Sex Union Is Endless When Breath Savoring*
        is the Only Way
        Anointing her body with unguents diverse—Bedecking
            her tresses with flowers
        fragrant—Do you enjoy the damsel in passion's union;—
            If your desire becomes
        devotion—Prana will shoot up through the Spinal
            Pathway—
        Then your enjoyment is endless.

826. *If Breath is Savored, Delicious Enjoyment Results in*
        Erotic Union
        When they seek enjoyment—The breath standeth still;—
            The full breasted damsel

---

*In order to fathom the Sringara profundities of Khajuraho, one would need to *feel* the sustained reverential awe of looking at the ceiling of the Sistine Chapel but with the ars erotica Khajuraho images painted there—looking with humbled and transformed amazement without wavering back to the scientia sexualis perspectives at all. For more on Khajuraho, see http://indiaouting.com/files/2011/07/3.jpg and http://indiaouting .com/files/2011/07/6.jpg.

†On the myriad compromising vicissitudes—patriarchy, elitist popular cultural hierarchies, "gotta make a living somehow" pressures, and more—in the history of Indian erotic tantra, see David Gordon White, *Kiss of the Yogini.*

and fervent male—Stand in union exalted;—As liquid
   silver and gold—Their
passions emissions—In rapture commingleth.

827. *Duration of Enjoyment Lengthens If Breath is Savored*
   in the Copulatory
   Yoga That is Practiced By the Hero and the Heroine—
   Upward they drive the coach of breath—
   That has its wheels in regions right and left;—
   There they collect the waters of the heaven—And never
   the organs tiring know.

828. *Xylemic Upflowing of Semen Urdhvaretas Through*
   Breath Savoring—
   This is the Meaning of That Union;
   When in the sex act semen prepares to liquefy—
   The yogi xylemic feels Seed turn instead into heart's
   golden devotion to Goddess—
   And attains urdhvaretas depths within;—And a
   matured auras radiator he then becomes.

829. *Effect of Xylemic Upward Savoring of Urdhvaretas*
   Xylemic Flow
   He becomes fully matured of Knowing the path to all—
   the Enjoyment of all—
   He becomes fully matured of self—He becomes fully
   matured of senses five.

830. *Sex Union Through the Pariyanga Lasts Five Ghatikas*
   and is Bliss
   This is Pariyanga Yoga (cot yoga)—That lasts five
   ghatikas (2 hours)
   Beyond the sixth—The damsel sleeps in the arms of the
   lover
   Whom she has worshipped, too—In union blissful
   That fills the heart—And passes description.

831. *Matured Urdhvaretas Attainers Alone Can Resort to*
   Pariyanga

Unless it be,—He had matured in urdhvaretas—The
Pariyanga yoga—
Of five ghatikas length—No yogi/yogini shall—A
woman/man embrace . . . .
834. *Only Those Who Have Attained Khecari Puberty Have*
the Maturity for Pariyanga
Lest the silvery liquid into the golden flow,—The artful
goldsmiths (practitioner)
sealed and savored it up with yogic breath—The sparks
(Kundalini) that flew traveled up
by way of Spinal tube—There above,—They contained
them with tongue's tip.[1]

Within the yogic cosmology of reincarnation and antara-bhavas, these twilight teachings hold that Sringara Rasa is the most matured of all "enlightenment realms," enjoyed literally "in heaven," between earthly births. Or do these teachings refer to an earthly Sringara Rasa, as well? Perhaps the Sringara realm is permeated by *samsara,* the struggles, tragedies, and even horrors of human life, here and now, not in a fantasied utopian future? Indeed, perhaps as the neo-teachers teach and live, there is no urdhvaretas, no "authentic yoga," no brahmacharya saints, no God/Goddess, and no limitations within a "scientia sexualis" to even be concerned about; heaven is simply, "Be-Here-Now."

Or (as I believe), does Sringara Rasa emerge in its fullest glory only in wisely hidden, "beyond the pale" esoteric circles surrounding a living saint, such as Thirumoolar, whose shaktipat energies radiate from the vibrations of the twilight and kavi-poetic text as much as, or more than, from the semantic purport of the verses, vibrations that awaken and nurture the khechari prerequisite within this mystical *mandala* or "circle of initiates?" If so, perhaps it is because we are also in a dark wintery cosmic season that began in the Iron Age, the *Kali Yuga,* that is slowly shifting inexorably into the spring era of an approaching next myriad thousands of years of *Dvapara Yuga* when charismatic ars eroticas of all sorts will once again (as they have countless times before in previous yuga cyclings) break through the world's many reductive scientia sexualises and spontaneously emerge for the whole world family, like green buds after a "long, cold lonely winter"?[2]

BEYOND PROTECTIVE AMBIGUITIES
AND SCHOLARLY DEMYSTIFYING CERTAINTIES
INTO THE SACRED INTIMUS

When your lifelong loyal love relationship has traversed from cynical and scientia sexualis certainties into ever more sustained living in evanescent subtleties and the intimus, when you and your lifelong loyal love partner have reunited love-lust-fertility-devotion-play into an all-blended-together wholeness nurturing perineum-to-pineal maturity, when you have attained fluency with emotional and verbal communication and problem solving, and when you have opened access to numerous Inner Empathic Spaces, then you will be living at the entranceway to Sringara Rasa, the "heaven" of matured ars erotica passions. Khajuraho, Tibetan Buddhism Yab-Yum tangkas, and all pariyanga texts will be accessible to your ars erotically matured eyes, flowing with ecstatic tears of recognition, beyond the scholar's puzzles, new age nascent understandings, and the psychoanalyst's polymorphic distortions.

When the beauty of life and the great expanse of the tongue-awakened, perineum to pineal khecari puberty has blossomed, lovers' devotional kisses, anywhere and everywhere, include a drinking of each other's secreted entheogenic madhu nectars whose consciousness-enhancing powers derive from unlocking the matured creativity of retas, the seeds of life itself. These beyond semen, beyond ova, seed of seed nectars imbibed, through every pore and via visually "drinking each other in," with speaking and hearing in endless repartees of "Om, Honey," responded to with "Om, Baby," responded to together with "We have found the endless way," will nourish the rasas of ever-deeper devotion that provoke the curtains of the body to part and reveal yet another delicious realm of Holy of Holies and powerful aphrodisiacal nectars, as Melanie and Renee glimpsed.

We were tasting each other in a closeness we prefer to not tell you about, except to say that I felt like I was on acid or MDMA because Melanie became so wondrous to me, I can only compare it with a drug trip, but we don't even drink! She was my goddess and I was hers. But it was "just us," not something new agey at all. First, it was like total empathy for our whole life of suffering and all the years of breakups we went through, like a willingness to literally drink in each other's darkest sweaty struggles, to know each other deeply. There were tears, and we licked them off each other with great tenderness. But then we got sweeter and sweeter to one another, higher and higher. We were getting free from every one of our sexual fears, hopes, and concerns, we were "worshipping" everything about each other, then endlessly dancing with each other. I try to explain it to you now, but you'd have to have been there, if you know what I mean. It's been a year and we've never shared anything like it since. It was just a perfect storm of perfect us, a taste of heaven, ha! for a while.

Lifelong loyal love is the bond required by and further strengthened by these admixing exchanges of the silvery and golden bodily elixirs of life. As Xun Liu notes regarding Taoist pariyanga of duo-cultivation, there must be "genuine rapport" and mutual lifelong respect between the partners without which "the Phoenix does not chirp and the Turtle will not rise."[3]

The twenty-year retas project, begun ideally by couples in their mid to late twenties, of creatively raising children to adulthood (and of elder care of parents and grandparents) can also bestow couples with the maturity requisite to approach Sringara Rasa. Thus, in their mid to late fifties, after the children have left the nest, the grihasthin couple has the time and foundation to extend their personal yoga sadhanas and couples' practice periods and go forth into the longer hours of Sringara Rasa unions, beyond the pale of daily life schedules and concerns. As noted earlier, childless couples' spiritual growth requires creative projects for our world family that are "equal to" raising a child or two, even for those living simple lives of private contentment. There are no shortcuts, no mere "be here now" consciousness shifts that skip us over this broad foundation of full maturation. Here are three more glimpses into Sringara Rasa from my couples work.

Frank: Once we got that eight-year thorn out of my foot of the affair or whatever the hell it was, then there wasn't anything in the way for us. Our house had always been where all the kids came over to hang out with our kids, pancake breakfasts for twenty or thirty of them the morning of the big high school football games, everybody cracking jokes, including those kids from broken homes, the "lost puppies" we would call them, and we could've been one of them, seriously, that's how close we got to it those years with that sliver gnawing at me that had broken our perfection; yeah, all along we have been best friends, best lovers, best parents. And I am a big guy, coach of the team and all that, so when I cried like a lost baby in Caroline's arms and she started crying too, somehow, we got free and it all came together. I don't want anything more, why should I? It's all here, and we are ready to learn more, we will be your best students, I guarantee it!

Susan to Andrew: You just taste amazing! And your touch makes me feel how amazing I am; I didn't know that before, none of this! And even though we got separated for about three years, I couldn't think of anyone else but you, and here we are, and all we went through since then! We have our oasis and it's always right there, endlessly there, no matter what else has to be taken care of. It's perfect!

Natalia (translated from Russian): You talked about rasas and all that was kind of interesting, but it didn't really do it for us. When you merely said, "Worship each other with every touch, every lick, and word," that worked for us. Now we are there. Spaceba, Stuart.

Another aspect of Sringara Rasa is all heart, soul to soul and transcends the erotic-romantic and the physical realm entirely, as we see in this moving client vignette of a Down syndrome man and his brother that "just happened."

Michael: I was watching Erich from across the room as he was watching TV and all of a sudden all of his Down features evaporated and in the exact moment that his face came into perfect focus, Erich jumped out of his chair, made a beeline to me, and threw his arms around me and said, "I love you, Michael," and then he turned around and went back to his chair. He felt me see him, that's what it was.

And here is another glimpse, beyond the pale, hidden and revealed in the twilight language that could not be any clearer but, then, "you'd have to be there."

Mouths are inner-domed temples of echo-chambered yearning, wedding altars for entheogenic transubstantiations of each other's honey-madhu sentience that wax and wane with the retas cycling lunar orb. Tongues are saints in their oral pulpits crying ars erotic love songs. Genitals are Holiest of Holies, magnetizing all with retas powers, blood cells jubilant with laughter, partners glued forever. In the moment of such unions, all devils cower as their dark loneliness is healed, all angels a-million trilling, every cell awake and quivering, spirituality charismatica, the endless wedding feast. Lifelong loyal love, the only truth there is.

And here is a scene from a story (or is it a true account?), entitled "Spiritual Wealth" by Baba Hari Dass, about the quietly meditative brahmacharya couple, Sulochana and her husband, Ramdeen.

Year after year passed and they both remained in the same cave, sitting in silence and enjoying the calmness of the jungle. They began to feel that they didn't need to use words or talk to each other because they knew each other's thoughts very well. All their communication was done through their mental waves, whether they were sitting together or far apart physically.

Ramdeen explained how this connection came about in this way:

Once long ago, my wife was sitting here all alone while I was sitting outside somewhere. She heard a sound inside her head. The sound became louder and louder. When I entered the cave I saw her sitting with her eyes closed, with no body consciousness. I rushed to her and tried to see if she was alive, but when my head touched hers, at once the sound started in my head, too. . . . After that, we don't know what happened . . . when we came to our senses, we felt a peace which can't be described . . . we sit in this cave and listen to that sound which . . . spreads all over the body . . . coming out through the pores of the skin and vibrates inside this cave . . . [now] for us the whole world is a cave and a jungle.

Baba Hari Dass continues:

The cave was changed into a big temple . . . but no one knows what happened to Ramdeen and Sulochana. Are they living in an invisible body?[4]

13
Brahmacharya

Solo Intimacy with the Source

The most well-known advanced aspects
of primordial gender worship
have occurred internally within the person of a
*   singular body*
surrendering alone to the longings for God
(Christ in the desert, Buddha under his tree,
*   En-caved Shiva)*
to know for sure, without end,
to feel bliss and love supreme,
to activate all gendered powers,
to revere all, forgive all, mature all, to conquer
*   death*
attaining samadhi realization,
all retas powers of a thousand children's children
completely activated—"gone all the way"
from origin-most source to blossom-most fruition,
All seed-fuel burned—nirbija—to vibhuti ashes
*   exhausted*
with no private ego reserves, the end of trepid
*   longing*
and the beginning of yet other realms supreme.

Would you like to spend your life helping the neediest of the needy, living simply yourself, with numerous hours per day for yogic worship, thus fathoming the yoga of all the great yogis of yore, feeling deepest kinship with them? Does *caritas* heart caring and compassionate love move you so much more than any of the many moods of erotica, to the extent that you passionately want to serve humanity as much as you can?

Are you in love with the simple, solitary spiritual life, but don't want to join a monastery or ashram, or perhaps you would love that, too? Do you want to live the ancient yogic way, then teach yoga or lead kirtan or study Sanskrit from these depths? Do you want to know what the ancient texts really mean? Are Mother Kundalini's energies coursing through you and you wonder how to best proceed and are single?

Does melting every seed and desirous power of the genital puberty and of all gender possibilities into every dimension of your being without a trace of scientia sexualis aspirations for erotic partners or other "sexual" simulations "turn you on"?

Is the universe calling you to run off with Her, leave it all behind and elope with Her, live and die and merge with Her and Her alone?

Is God/Goddess so real for you that He/She is all you think about? Are scriptures and theologies, myths and philosophies all you ever really want to read? Are Christ, Mary, Buddha, St. Francis, Teresa d'Avila, Hildegard von Bingen, Meister Eckhart, Shiva, Parvati, Amma-ji, Ramana, Nityananda, Thich Nhat Hanh, Kripalvananda, Baba Hari Dass, and company not merely heroes for you, but arm-in-arm brethren to you?

Don't worry about the judgments of others about your "arrogance." I understand you only too deeply: the humility and naturally compelling simplicity from which you so identify with the saints of all times is the farthest thing from arrogance. I affirm what you are drawn to—to live solo brahmacharya with love's full abandon, to live the "spiritual life" of the ages—as do fifty million of your brethren and sisters throughout all history and cultures. You may be solitary, but you are not alone.

Are gods of all religions your favorite conversation topic, a love never diminished by any scientific agnosticism, church or guru scandals, psychoanalytic reductionism, or even popular "nondual" eliminations of a God above, or any other dissuasions to "believing" of all times? Or perhaps the impersonal humbled perfection calls you "beyond yourself."

Are all these enticements so great that the chapters on family creation and the daily life challenges and loves of grihastha, and even the heat that smolders within Sringara Rasa conjugal X-rated pariyanga, fade into a realm for others, but not for you?

If so, all gods and goddesses rejoice your well-understood initiation into profound brahmacharya urdhvaretas inner marriage. Not a second to waste, Lord is there, so enter with shuddering awe, ego-quelling humility, and ominous profundity into the simplicity of solo brahmacharya life. Here are some indications of how that might manifest.

Serene as a mirror-surfaced pond, an hour before dawn. The ethereally shifting darkness calls you awake with the pulling feeling of the imminent barely glimmering sunrise and your body magnetically arises like a flower effortlessly being turned toward the sun. You leave your bed, which is needed only six or eight hours, anyway, a simple resting place and no more. Something more thrilling than more minutes of sleep always calls you to your yoga shrine: a six-by-eight never-stepped-upon sheepskin covering a two-inch foam pad for your spontaneous yoga. This is ars erotica yoga of being moved *and you need such a protective shrine on which to unfold.*

As dawn emerges, sun and moon writhe together at the base of your spine, sending sun goddess Gayatri up your spine, radiating out all your spinal nerves. Thus, after your ablutions, your yogic dance begins from within every DNA strand to every longing toward yoga, union. Om Shiva Shakti Ma! Practice pranayama for as long as you like, singing-chanting-dancing, shifting through various moods of devotion from minor-chord longings to joyous laughter, as arise from your heart of hearts. Meditation for as long as you like. Gratitude . . . you have made devotion to yoga your centermost. Every day you "get to love yoga," chanting with heart-searing and consolidating devotion, something like this: "Yoga, you are my mother, my father, my spouse, my children, my friend, retas is blossoming in earnest in me, through thick and think, we are One!"

And what about the rest of your day? Most likely, you will be inspired to apply your skills and passions to the greatest needs of humanity. Income becomes pure pragmatics, enough to pay the bills. As you mature, various *siddhis* (spiritual or psychic powers), ethical purities, compassions, and creative abilities can emerge to help you master ever more complex projects; you might need project money, and it might come to you in great abundance. Then and always, utmost ethicality with money, work, and the treatment of all is essential. You always know that your priceless treasures cannot be purchased, so what care do you have for material luxuries? Authority and power might also come your way; take care to use it to empower others and to represent the truths that are solutions based in one world family, lifelong relationships, and your own balance between work, yoga, and goofing off.

See issues from all points of view, liberal to conservative, ars erotica to scientia sexualis, the wealthy, the middle, and the poor economic groups, and on and on, beyond simple allegories and categories of good guys and bad guys, yet find your way into the actions you are then moved to take. Leading all, following all—quietly and anonymously or dramatically and center staged—toward harmonies of closeness, attuned to the most accurate facts and well-defined truths or intuited and time-honored principles you know.

Flirtation is for others, though others might be allured by you more than you realize. You are a yogi. You walk among all with yoga as your monogamous, true-blue sweetie and beloved. So you arrive home each night, perhaps enjoy a soiree with beloved yoga for some time, then zoom into surrendered sleep early enough to again awaken predawn for more, more, more beloved yoga, touching Lord's hem, allowing Her to dance you toward asanas, mudras of hands, eyes, tongue, voice, mind.

Your urethra may become self-rejuvenating in xylemic, inward-drinking vajroli mudra, with retas streaming from your hypothalamus, pineal, ovaries/testes throughout your whole body, into manipura chakra, alluring Kundalini. Then no energies or scientia sexualis images or possibilities will tether you to "the worldly" world. Urdhvaretas will radiate ever more wildly into bursts of light, bliss, laughter, awesome beatitudes of tumescent stillness. The world you live in glows ethereal like moonlight, with retas fecundity. You are unshakably a yogi, shaken only by Ma!

If possible, spend some months each year in India, far beyond modern ways that are saturated with scientia sexualis. Visit matured urdhvaretas yogis whenever possible. Seek shaktipat blessings, should you feel spiritual connection with one of them. Be open to "everything will change," whereby your yoga only deepens. Learn Sanskrit; fast regularly; sing often; hold no grudge, seek no fame.

> On that joyous night,
> In secret, seen by no one,
> Nor with anything in sight,
> I had no other light or mark,
> Than the one burning in my heart.
>
> St. John of the Cross,
> "Dark Night"[1]

THE HEIGHTS

The heights by great men reached and kept were not attained by sudden flight, but they, while their companions slept, were toiling upward in the night.

Longfellow,
"The Ladder of St. Augustine"

What are these heights that only profound yogis know? A brief quote from Kripalvananda's commentary on the *Hatha Yoga Pradipika,* a central ars erotica yogic text from the fifteenth century, gives us a glimpse into them, toward where you are hourly, daily, by the decade, maturing:

Anatomically, there are three uvulas in the body. Each stands at the entrance of a three-path convergence, where two gross physical side paths and one (dorsal, back) subtle energy central path meet to form a lower path. The first uvula is, in a female body, the *external os*, the part of the cervix of the uterus projecting into the vagina. The two longer sides of the uterus lead up to the uterine tubes and the ovaries. In a male body, the first uvula is a small eminence projecting into the urethral orifice, just above the prostatic utricle, where the two *ductus deferens* branch upward on their way to the testes. The second uvula is the part of the soft palate that hangs down at the back of the mouth at the back entrance to the nasal cavity, with its two internal nasal openings, which is of the same tissue type as the anterior (front) lobe of the pituitary gland. This uvula can be elevated, by swallowing or by the throat lock, to block the nasal cavity. The third uvula is situated between the two hemispheres (tonsils) of the cerebellum near the choroid plexus of the fourth ventricle. From it, two main nerve pathways from the dorsal part of the central canal of the spinal cord pass to the higher centers of the brain, including the posterior (rear) lobe of the pituitary, the hypothalamus, the pineal gland, the choroid plexus of the third ventricle, and the cerebrum.

If, by abandonment of attachment, and openness to divinity, the sexual seed and the life energy are prevented at that point from falling down into the lower path, the seed is absorbed into the blood and the energy goes up the central path [past the first, second and third uvuli]. The greater the degree of detachment and surrender to God, the higher up the seed and the energy are held, the more the seed evolves and the more subtle the energy grows, and the more stable both become. In the end, both the physical body and the life energy are absorbed into divinity, and the *yogi* is in his natural [fully matured of all potentials] state.[2]

THE SAINT

The most matured solo urdhvaretas saint that I have come across was documented in Baba Hari Dass's *Hariakhan Baba: Known, Unknown;* Govindan's *Babaji;* and Satyeswarananda's *Babaji,* each maintaining that Hariakhan Baba, manifester of many siddhis, was the candle-to-candle initiator of Neem Karoli Baba, popularly known as the "mind-reading guru" of Richard Alpert (Ram Dass). He was of the lineage of Paramahansa Yogananda, one of the first yogis to come to the West at the turn of the century. Yogananda attained additional esteem after his death in 1952 when, with some controversy, his corpse showed no signs of decomposition, even after some twenty days, according to the notarized statement of Los Angeles Mortuary Director H. T. Rowe.

> The absence of any visual signs of decay in the dead body of Paramahansa Yogananda offers the most extraordinary case in our experience . . . . No physical disintegration was visible in his body even twenty days after death. . . . No indication of mold was visible on his skin, and no visible desiccation (drying up) took place in the bodily tissues. This state of perfect preservation of a body is, so far as we know from mortuary annals, an unparalleled one. . . . No odor of decay emanated from his body at any time . . . There is no reason to say that his body had suffered any visible physical disintegration at all.[3]

According to the late Vinit-muni of Pransali, India, Hariakhan Baba/Babaji might also be (or be related to) Lakulisha (150 CE–circa 1955! Or ?), who initiated Swami Kripalvananda (whose corpse showed no signs of *rigor mortis* during the two days before his burial in the early 1950s, (and perhaps many other unknown yogis).[4] According to Collins, Lakulisha's image remains embossed in the Ellora Kailash and Elephanta Island carvings (dated 500–600 CE), which point to the practice of kundalini yoga as "the origin and culmination of all life."[5] The *Vayu Purana,* the *Kurma Purana,* and the *Linga Purana* discern Lakulisha or Nakulisha as the purported twenty-eighth incarnation of Shiva, Lord of Yoga. In his erudite *The Alchemical Body,* scholar David G. White also describes Lakulisha as the touchstone authenticator of numerous successive legendary yogis.

According to the *Pashupata Sutra* and the *Ganakarika Sutra,* the Lakulisha Kundalini yoga sect practiced an ecstatic ritual, including wild laughter, sacred singing, "dancing consisting of [all possible] motions of the hands and feet: upward, downward, inward, outward and shaking motion," a sacred "sound produced by the contact of the tongue-tip with the palate . . . after the dance when the devotee has again sat down and is still meditating on Siva," an "inner worship," and "prayer."[6] I suggest that such dancing and singing were not mere merriment, but were sahaja or charismatic shaktipat manifestations that were codified into standardized asanas, mudras, and bandhas.

This Shakta-Shaivite revival spread massively throughout Hindu, Buddhist, and Jain India for some 600 years, producing one of the greatest outpourings of temple construction in human history. The sect was noteworthy in Indian history for its belief in a deity capable of bestowing redemptive grace beyond the causal dictates of karma.

Lakulisha and his followers believed (as did the original Franciscan cult) that, as forest-dwelling yogis, they transformed the strife of city dwellers by absorbing social ridicule or by receiving homage and bestowing shaktipat blessings upon the populace. Indeed, the prejudices of caste and other animosities evaporated during their shaktipat rituals through collective initiation into the deepest intimacies of ars erotica life.

ELDER SANNYASA, LETTING GO

For older couples the grihastha path unfolds its long-developing passion and attains its golden auric climax only after a lifetime of sharing.

Chandra, seventy-five, and Raj, seventy-eight, have been married for fifty-two years. Their lives have been busy with dual careers and family life. "Too busy for a midlife crisis," says Raj. Since they are "basically celibate," they take up the later-life brahmacharya of their Indian ancestors known as sannyasa, the world-shedding stage of life. After their meditations and prayers, they tearfully share their amazement at what now comes out of hiding from behind the decades of daily routines. Their children are all married, and now they are letting go into the Infinite, a little more each day, sometimes together, sometimes quite alone. They are making their ways from Here to There.

They embrace a schedule of hours each day for prayer, meditation, scriptures, walks (perhaps with walkers, someday, but not now!), family check-ins, and some volunteer mentoring. Life has gotten simpler and simpler. Even the aches, Raj's blindness, and other health issues don't upset them. "So it goes," is their favorite phrase in this "letting go" that gives them the peace of slowly vanishing their egoic striving each day into *Aum, Shanti, Shanti, Aum*. Their children look on, wistfully inspired, and feel blessed.

Afterword

The urdhvaretas map of human development shows how romantic-erotic love and marriages can grow for a whole lifetime with just as dramatic a pace as our personal maturation during our teen-puberty years, fostering the kind of lifelong relationships that then lead to loving, secure, unbroken family lineages, to be passed on generation upon generation, "as far as the eye can see."

Spiritual enlightenment itself becomes a fully embodied and generation-to-generation continuous and ever-expanding process of seed-infused radiance perhaps someday embracing the whole Vasudhaiva kutumbakam, culturally diverse world. For within urdhvaretas, there is always another fractal realm of retas potentials within another and another, which allure us inwardly ever closer to some mysteriously shared Origin of origins, Seed of all seeds realm, and outwardly toward the angelic beauty of every newborn, the budding radiance of every child and teen entering puberty aglow with matured seed-within-seed mysteries herself, every starry-eyed couple in love, each pregnant woman in contented wholeness, wide-eyed new father and brimming grandpa and grandma.

Indeed, when a Buddha "ends all rebirth" via his ecstatic inner marriage, this is the profound storehouse of powers he has "burned up" in order to do so. Consider what it would be like to awaken analogous, deeply resting, creative-retas powers in your own embodied life and relationships, now and forever forward. This is the matured "duality that approaches nonduality" that all saints guide us toward, one that has grown real roots in engaged, embodied living, roots that *hold* and verify our maturity and spiritual creativity. In its ever more flesh-permeating pathways, it breathes charismatic energies into us from the twilight ars erotica teachings of the great bhakti-kavi and tantric scriptures, as well.

Yet the scientia sexualis of mainstream Western religions and psychology have only given us garbled or fundamentally deseeded understandings of how the great seed powers, the prepotent soul of it all, can ever more fully radiate into our lives. The inner antidesire conflicts, familial brokenness, cynicisms, and shallow yet ubiquitous scientia prodesire eroticisms of modern culture perfectly reflect the exact ways those faulty maps are garbled and shallow. Their politics have turned deep mysteries of gender, fertility, reverence, and the passions of arousal into shrill debates that rest on these worn-out soils, pretending to be bedrock truths of life and freedom.

Nearly four decades ago, a two-thousand-year-old yogic candle-to-candle tradition extended its hand to me with love and tenderness, revealing a way beyond these broken times and onto ars erotica terra firma, just as I extend some few glimmers of its twilight radiances to you through this book. May these glowing seeds of love mature well and blossom in your own life, in the lives of those near and dear to you, and in our shared, One Family world.

Glossary

advaita: nonduality, a fully activated life of nuanced wisdom, qualified over the millennia in India as *dvaita-advaita,* dual-and-nondualism, to highlight nuance-discerning powers and to accommodate ethics, values, and variances such as *ardhanari* (half male, half female), then/now/later, God/demigod/guru/human, and eras including golden-eras-of-fullness (*sat-yuga*) and eras-progressing-toward-or-away-from-fullness (*dvarapa, treta,* and *kali yugas*); all such distinctions are typically lost in the popularized neo-advaita teachings on "nonduality."

ahamkara: self-sense, or ego, which can be isolated from the more subtle jiva, or soul, and thus becomes bereft of spiritual input and believes itself to be limited to the physical body.

ajna chakra (cakra): midbrow center of ultimate discernment and source of retas bliss of the endlessly consummating inner marriage.

amrita: immortality-ambrosia essence.

anahata chakra (cakra): heart center, associated with love and courage, presides over the air element and the prana-maya kosha; seat of "the unstruck" origin of the heartbeat, jiva and ahamkara.

anahata-nad: charismatic, "unstruck" or inspired emotional-development sound making or chanting.

ananda-maya kosha (kosa): bliss or causal body, where jiva dwells.

anna-maya kosha (kosa): food-eating body; the fleshy, physical body.

antara-bhavas: nonphysical, interbirth existence realms; *bardos* in Tibetan cosmology.

apana pran: pranic currents of abdomen concerned with elimination and reproductive/sexual functions.

ars erotica: Michel Foucault's term for erotic knowledge and practices focusing specifically on profundity of bodily pleasures, thus able to include sexual, meditative, mystical, and celibate pleasures and ecstasies and a wide range of "orgasms" and "unions."

asana: a formal position or pose in hatha yoga also termed "tumescences" in our study of sahaja yoga as an ars erotica.

atman: soul, the inmost seed essence of any being.

auras: golden-haloed or hallowed retas matured to saintly heights.

avandhana: enlightened learning-concentration-understanding capacities; learning taken to meditative depths wherein the siddhi of extraordinary intellectual cognition and memory can "awaken." Neo-meditative teachings regarding enlightenment based in exclusionary tropes of "beyond intellect" or "empty mind" will be greatly enriched as avandhana ars erotica meditation becomes more well known via masters such as Dr. R. Ganesh.

ayurveda: yogic system of medicine and physiology.

bandhas: muscular contractions, or "locks," that keep subtle energies in a specific area of the body for the purpose of healing and urdhvaretic maturation.

Bhagavad Gita: "Song of God," sermon on life from Krishna to Arjuna; usually understood as dealing with karma yoga, the ways of dutiful and honorable activity in the world.

bhakti yoga: the yoga based in deepening love and devotional feelings.

bindu: the essence of the gamete, sexual fluids, seed force.

brahmacharya (brahmacarya): moving or living in accord with absolute truths or god; yoga practice infused with the fertility seed energies of life and mind-body maturation known as *retas*, the physical connection with God via the power of life creation.

brahmarandhra: subtle center at the crown of the head attuned to absolute truths and ideals corresponding to ultimate reality.

buddhi: intellectual power of mind.

chakras (cakras): nonphysical energy centers that regulate the physical and more subtle bodies.

charismatics: "divine gifts" or spontaneously emergent ecstatic states that evoke siddhi powers and bodily "manifestations of the spirit" such as blissful-to-overwhelming bodily shaking of "being reborn" in many spiritual traditions, perhaps akin to maternal labor contractions.

cum: I have used *cum* to refer to maturational breakthroughs and fulfillments within the postgenital puberties of urdhvaretas and to "reclaim" and transform scientia sexualis terms for ars erotica purposes.

davening: Judaic prayer form accompanied by spinal-rocking, perhaps related to activated spinal energies.

dharana: near to complete unwavering concentration on an object.

dharma: a way, or manner, of life or of acting in a particular situation that is in accord with spiritual principles; virtuous or honorable living, which leads to the fullest maturation of the individual, the couple, the family, or the whole world family and planetary ecology.

dhyana: unwavering attention to an object; the beginning of meditation proper.

divya sharira (divya sarira): inwardly married, self-regenerating body of "divine light."

ekagrata: one-pointed concentration.

gopi: a devotee of bhakti yoga's god of love, Krishna, all of whom are "feminine" within ars erotica semantics, as distinct from scientia sexualis categories of gender.

grihastha: The adult stage of life of marriage and retas-family creation.

guru: "light that dispels darkness"; an enlightened teacher of yoga and dharma.

ha-tha (hatha) yoga: actions, practices, and transfixing tumescences that purify and mature the anna-, prana-, mano- and vijnana-maya koshas through urdhvaretas activation of developmental seed processes. Esoterically *ha-tha* is "sun-moon."

hesychast: Inwardly married person within the Orthodox tradition, often followers of St. John of Sinai's *Ladder of Divine Ascent* scripture.

ida: the main lunar or cooling channel that crosses the central spinal sushumna at each of the first six chakras.

intimus: Latin for "within," "most interior"; root of the word *intimacy*.

Ishvara (Isvara): God, the Primordial Mover.

ithyphallic: tumescence of the penis arising in the spinal puberty outside of scientia sexualis categories but often reduced by translators to "fertility symbol" or "sexual arousal" (likewise, **ithy-breasted**, nipple tumescences).

jiva: the being that has the life; the soul of one's being that exists independent of bodily life.

Jnaneshvari (Jnaneshvar Gita): an interpretation of the *Bhagavad Gita* of particular relevance to kundalini yoga, the yoga of complete bodily maturation and energetic transformations by Sri Jnaneshvar, an attainer of physical regeneration and complete inner-marriage union.

kaivalya: separated from all illusions and resting in the natural state; eternal beatitude.

karezza: coitus interruptus.

karma: actions and potentials: their consequences or manifestations.

kavi: a spiritually inspired poet.

khechari mudra (khecari): advanced stage of urdhvaretas in which the tongue spontaneously moves back toward the palatial cavity of the head, the "reverse" of an early stage of oral, cranial, and lingual embryological development, as the body seeks the "taste of" its own procreative source.

koshas (kosas): sheaths or gradients of the human being.

kumbhaka: prolonged suspension of the breath on either the held-in breath or the exhaled and held-out breath.

kundalini: intelligent Mother energy that, when awakened from latency in muladhara chakra (and perhaps in the ajna chakra), matures all retas potentials toward fully embodied enlightenment.

lila: activity of the universe considered as divine play.

lingam: penis or any tumescent organ or certain subtle-body structures with male powers in consort with yoni female powers; cosmic arising up of all thallus prephallic forms.

madhu: retas matured to the quintessential "honey" or "mead" intoxicant of love-bliss.

maha-samadhi: great knowing of the source of consciousness at the time of physical death and approached during near-death experiences.

manipura chakra (cakra): navel center, governs physical body, presides over fire principle; associated with willful emotionalities.

mano-maya kosha: mental-emotional sheath.

mantra: sacred Sanskrit incantation, often producing specific vibrational effects in the physical and subtle bodies.

mudra: gesture or "delight tumescence" relating to puberties of perineum, genitals, heart, tongue, eyes, gesticulating fingers and hands, pineal, cerebrum, and mindspace.

muladhara chakra (cakra): spinal base center, resting place of Mother Kundalini after completion of gestation, presides over earth element, associated with instincts of physical survival.

murcha: "swoon," to be overcome with awe.

nabhan mudra (nabho): tumescence of curling the tongue back in the mouth so that the tip touches the soft palate.

nadis: subtle bodily channels, analogous to acupuncture meridians.

neo-tantra, neo-yoga, neo-advaita: popularizations of Indian ars erotica spiritual traditions shaped by scientia sexualis concerns.

nigune: spontaneous or inspired chanting in Judaic traditions.

nirbija-samadhi: fully matured consciousness with complete activation or "burning/exhausting completely to ash" (an esoteric reference to exhausted retas) of the reservoir of all human seed potentials.

niyama: guidances for positive actions and observances.

Nyasa: placing of subtle energy, anointment.

ojas: transmuted bindu; radiantly glowing bioenergy.

pariyanga: "boudoir yoga" as described by medieval-era South India yogi Thirumoolar.

pingala: solar energy channel weaving caduceus-like along the spinal sushumna channel in consort with the ida lunar channel, intersecting at each of the first six chakras.

prana: vital energy of life; vitality in the air, food, and water.

prana pran: currents of prana in chest concerned with breathing.

prana-maya kosha (kosa): vital energy sheath.

pranayama: control or savoring of breath, or prana; breathing practices.

pranotthana (prana-utthana): intensified or uplifted pranic activity during pregnancy, teen puberty, and consequent to shaktipat initiations; a precursor to kundalini awakening.

pratyahara: early stage of meditation in which focus is gathered from its more ordinary scatterings through the senses and through "mind chatter."

prema: unconditional love.

qawwali: Islamic chanting style known for its breakthroughs into inspired, quivering ecstasies.

rajas: female retas or seed energies substance.

rasa: juices of life, hormones, purely subjective emotional states, alchemical substances with entheogenic or siddhi-nourishing capacities as noted in rasa-yana, the lore of the rasas, and in the writings on aesthetics by Abhinava-gupta.

retas: vital juice current, procreative essence, "seed of seeds," the energetic precursor to gametes or seeds.

sabija-samadhi: highest meditative state, with remaining seeds of unactivated human potential.

sadhana: spiritual practices that gather virtue, awakenings of rare capacities, powers, and energy.

sadhu: a mendicant, inwardly married yogi.

sahaja: spontaneous or self-arising.

sahasrara chakra (cakra): crown chakra, beyond all elements; awakens into effulgent brilliance and divine knowledge; "thousand-petaled lotus."

samadhi: meditation with concentration unwaveringly gathered unto the source realm of consciousness itself.

samana pran: pranic current between navel and heart, concerned with digestion.

sat-chit-ananda: quintessence of blissful knowing of ananda-maya kosha consciousness.

scientia sexualis: Michel Foucault's term for erotic knowledge, mainly of the Catholic Church and Freudian-shaped modern "sexology of liberated desires," which conforms to moral codes of the former and scientific or "scientistic" principles of the latter. It includes liberal/conservative political ideologies, as well as research methods, including the confessional, the psychoanalytic interview, the laboratory and demographic study, and the diagnostic-nosological classification.

shakti (sakti): feminine-nuanced spiritual force always in interactive rapport with its masculine-nuanced correlate, analogous to numerous charismatic phenomena such as the Holy Ghost of Christianity.

Shakti (Sakti): the Hindu goddess of primal energy.

shakti chalani: the charismatic or willful "moving of the shakti within."

shaktipat (shakti-pata-diksha; sakti-pata-diksa): transmission of awakening energy from a guru to an aspirant as an initiation.

shamanica medhra: Literally, "quieting of the genitals/penis," functionally indicating states of maturity after or beyond genital puberty.

shambhavi (sambhavi) mudra: Puberty and tumescence of the eyes and sight; seeing of the divine radiances and deities within and without.

Shiva (Siva): the Hindu deity who presides over yogis; an enlightened attainer of complete kundalini and urdhvaretas maturity is termed an "incarnation of Shiva."

shraddha (sraddha): faith.

shukra (sukra): male retas seed energies substances.

siddhi: any highly developed human capacity that so far exceeds cultural norms as to be termed a spiritual or psychic "power," such as healing, empathy to the point of "mind reading," entheogenic gnosis, nuanced discernment, extreme longevity, omniscience, and bodily transformations.

soma rasa: deity ambrosia essence.

Sringara rasa: lustful erotic interactivity matured to "heavenly" or enlightened levels of endless and wide-ranging nuances and interactive synchronies born of highly matured retas potentials.

sushumna: central spinal channel entwined by ida and pingala, through which kundalini processes proceed.

svadhisthana chakra (svadhishthana cakra): associated with sexual and reproductive functioning; presides over the water element.

talu (taluka): subtle energy gateway on soft palate where the reversed tongue in nabhan and khechari mudras helps preserve amrita and helps quiet the mind.

tantra: yoga of weaving the spiritual into the physical.

tapas: the ardor of sustained selfless, heat-purifying passion.

tejas: electrical brilliance.

Thxiasi num: Bushman term for spiritually transformative inner heat generated in meditative trance and spontaneous "dance," as in pranotthana or kundalini of yoga traditions.

udana pran: pranic currents from the throat to the top of the head; govern swallowing movements of throat and tongue.

uju kaya: upward-held body and straight-spine meditative sitting position that is seen as naturally occurring tumescences of the spine within ars erotica traditions and as willfully maintained straight-backed sitting in the disciplined meditative traditions.

urdhvaretas: upward-growing refinement or maturation of the seeds of life.

vairagha (vairagya): nonattachment arising from contentment and dispassion.

vajroli mudra: urethral puberty wherein natural "xylem-like" upward flow of retas energizes all other ars erotica puberties of spine, tongue, hypothalamus, pineal, all acting synergistically together, but typically hidden in penile or vaginal mechanico-techniques in yogic and Taoist texts and their translations.

vasana: subtle basis of desires.

vijnana-maya kosha (kosa): intellect sheath, capable of reflective knowing.

virya: a quintessential distillate of sublimation, arising from virtuous activity, as noted by Sri Aurobindo.

vishuddha chakra (cakra): throat center, presides over the etheric element; associated with the spirit of words.

viyoga: the hidden union that occurs when one believes that only separation exists, felt as "longing" of bhakti yoga, expressed in gestures, asanas, poetry, and chanting and in a wide range of love relationships.

vritti (vrtti): thought waves or intentions.

vyana pran: circulatory pranic currents that pervade the whole body.

vyutthana: "resurrect," to surrender in sustained, breathless, transfixed awe into the yoni mudra realm where all awareness "is born," to the point of near-death, and then to "rearise" into a wizened and matured knowing of the life-death juncture and Source. The transitional state in between one distinct state of consciousness or embodiment and another wherein temporarily "everything changes."

xylem: upward flow of plant rasas from roots through stems, toward leaves and flowers.

yama: moral guidance of moderation and restraint.

yoga: actions, moods, or sustained attainments that are in harmony or union with the deepest energies of human maturation and evolution.

yoni: nurturing womb source of all beings, encompassing vulva, vagina, and uterus, but with ars erotica metaphysical significance.

yoni mudra: the fertile, sentient-womb-space in which living bodies fructify and consciousness itself emerges from its "mysterious," scintillating precursors, deified as "gods/goddesses."

zikr: Islamic prayer form often involving ecstatic states and spinal rocking in Sufi traditions.

Notes

PROLOGUE. URDHVARETAS

1. Foucault, *The History of Sexuality,* 57–58.
2. *Bhagavad Gita* 7.11, as interpreted by the author.

CHAPTER 1. EVERYTHING WILL CHANGE

1. Foucault, *The History of Sexuality,* 159.
2. Krishna, *Kundalini: Path to Higher Consciousness,* 6–7.
3. Sara Davidson, "Ram Dass Has a Son! But Has This Revelation Changed His Conception of Love?" www.huffingtonpost.com/sara-davidson/ram-dass-has-a-son_b_777452.html.
4. India: "Divorce Rate in India," www.divorcerate.org/divorce-rate-in-india.html; "India Moves to Make it Easier for Couples to Divorce," www.bbc.co.uk/news/10284416, June 2010; "Divorce Rates of the World," www.nitawriter.wordpress.com/2007/04/04/divorce-rates-of-the-world, April 4, 2007, with chart showing India as lowest in the world at 1.1% but rapidly increasing in urban centers. Tibet: T. Zhang, "Marriage and Family Patterns in Tibet," *China Population Today* 14, nos. 3–4 (August 1997): 9. Navajo: Jones Payne Group, Inc. "Phase II Housing Needs Assessment and Demographic Analysis," Navajo People, 2008. United States: "Compare Divorce and Family Laws," http://divorce-laws.findthebest.com; "Divorce After 50 Grows More Common," www.nytimes.com/2013/09/22/fashion/weddings/

260

divorce-after-50-grows-more-common.html, September 20, 2013; "The Changing American Family," www.nytimes.com/2013/11/26/health/families.html, November 25, 2013; "Second, Third Marriages: Divorce Rates Explained," www.huffingtonpost.com/2012/03/06/second-third-marriages-divorce-rate_n_1324496.html, March 6, 2012. See also "Marriage, Family, & Stepfamily Statistics," www.smartstep families.com/view/statistics, March 2013; "Is Serial Monogamy Worth Pursuing?" www.psychologytoday.com/blog/in-the-name-love/200810/is-serial-monogamy-worth-pursuing, October 31, 2008.

CHAPTER 2. ENTERING THE MYSTERY

1. Rendered from the ancient yogic text *Hatha Yoga Pradipika*, 1.40–43.

CHAPTER 3. SHARED-GENDER MYSTERY

1. Buber, *I and Thou*, 4.
2. Wittgenstein, *Philosophical Investigations*, 8.

CHAPTER 4. PURPOSEFUL URDHVARETAS

1. Aurobindo and the Mother, *On Love*, 10–11.
2. Marty Balin, *Crown of Creation* album (EMI Music Publishing, Universal Music Publishing Group, 1968).
3. Saint-Exupéry, *The Little Prince*, 83.
4. Ibid.
5. Ibid., 87.
6. Valerie Simpson and Nickolas Ashford (EMI Music Publishing, 1966).

CHAPTER 5. YOGIC ANATOMY AND TRANSFORMATION OF THE ARS EROTICA BODY

1. Vyas Dev, *Science of Soul*, 225.
2. Mitchell, *Bhagavad Gita*, 11.3–6.
3. Ramanujan, *Speaking of Siva*, 168.
4. Dass and Aparna, *The Marriage and Family Book*, 66.

5. Jnaneshvari, *Jnaneshvari*, 129, 132–33.
6. Woodroffe, *Principles of Tantra*, xiii.
7. Money, *Love and Love Sickness*, 119.
8. Kadloubovsky and Palmer, *Writings from the Philokalia*, 33.

CHAPTER 6. COMMITMENT AND MARRIAGE AS GRIHASTHA MYSTERIES

1. Saint-Exupéry, *The Little Prince*, 84.

CHAPTER 7. THE PASSIONS AND MYSTERIES OF FERTILITY

1. Masters, Johnson, and Kolodny, *Masters and Johnson on Sex and Human Loving*, 558.

CHAPTER 10. RELATIONAL WORSHIP

1. George Harrison, "Mystical One" (Umlaut Corporation, 1982).
2. Ramakrishnan, *Who Is Meher Baba?*, 120.
3. Sovatsky, "Clinical Forms of Love Inspired by Meher Baba's Mast Work," 135.
4. Kripalvananda via Joel Feldman, http://tinyurl.com/mzgdjjy, January 4, 2014.

CHAPTER 11. HATHA YOGA AS ARS EROTICA

1. Kripalvananda, *Science of Meditation*, 171–72.
2. Brooks et al., *Meditation Revolution*, 36.

CHAPTER 12. SRINGARA RASA

1. Adapted from B. Natarajan's translation of Thirumoolar's *Thirumandiram*.
2. George Harrison, "Here Comes the Sun" (Apple Records, 1969).

3. Liu, "Numinous Father and Holy Mother," 128.

4. Dass, *Sweeper to Saint,* 124–39.

CHAPTER 13. BRAHMACHARYA

1. de Nicolás, *St. John of the Cross,* 103.

2. Kripalvananda, *Revealing the Secret,* 163.

3. Yogananda, *Autobiography of a Yogi,* 575.

4. Kripalvananda, *Guru Prasad.*

5. Collins, *The Iconography and Ritual of Siva at Elephanta,* 48.

6. Ibid., 137–38.

Bibliography

American Catholic. "St. Thomas Aquinas." www.americancatholic.org/features/saints/saint.aspx?id=1274 (accessed March 3, 2014).

American Psychiatric Association. *Diagnostic and Statistical Manual of Mental Disorders DSM-IV-R).* 4th ed. Washington, DC: American Psychiatric Association, 1994. (5th ed., 2013)

Anand, Margot. *The Art of Sexual Ecstasy: The Path of Sacred Sexuality for Western Lovers.* Los Angeles: Jeremy P. Tarcher, 1990.

Aranya, Swami Hariharananda. *Yoga Philosophy of Patanjali.* Translated by P. N. Mukerji. Albany: State University of New York Press, 1983.

Arenson, David. "A Life of Celibacy—Revelation, Suffering, or Gateway to Higher Experience?" *Elephant Journal,* September 21, 2012. www.elephantjournal.com/2012/09/a-life-of-celibacy-revelation-suffering-or-gateway-to-higher-experience (accessed December 23, 2013).

Ariès, Philippe. *Western Attitudes toward Death from the Middle Ages to the Present.* Translated by Patricia Ranum. Baltimore: Johns Hopkins University, 1974.

Arnold, Edward A., ed. *As Long as Space Endures: Essays on the Kalacakra Tantra in Honor of H. H. the Dalai Lama.* Ithaca, N.Y.: Snow Lion Publications, 2009.

Aurobindo, Sri, and The Mother. *On Love.* Pondicherry, India: Sri Aurobindo Ashram, 1973.

Avalon, Arthur [Sir John Woodroffe]. *The Serpent Power: The Secrets of Tantric and Shaktic Yoga.* New York: Dover, 1974.

Axis Mundi. "Anahata-nad Kundalini Chanting." www.soundclick.com/ axismundi (accessed December 23, 2013).

Baba, Meher. *Hazrat Babajan.* Poona, India: Meher Era Publication, 1998.

Baker, Lynn S. *The Fertility Fallacy: Sexuality in the Post-Pill Age.* Philadelphia: Saunders Press, 1981.

Barbach, Lonnie. *For Yourself: The Fulfillment of Female Sexuality.* Garden City, N.Y.: Anchor, 1976.

Barrel, J. "Sexual Arousal in the Objectifying Attitude." *Review of Existential Psychology and Psychiatry* 8, no. 1 (1974).

Bentov, Itzhak. "Micromotion of the Body as a Factor in the Development of the Nervous System." In Lee Sannella, *Kundalini: Psychosis or Transcendence?* San Francisco: Dakin, 1977.

Bhagavad Gita: A New Translation. Translated by Stephen Mitchell. New York: Harmony Books, 2000.

Bion, Wilfred. *Transformations: Change from Learning to Growth.* New York: Basic Books, 1965.

Blake, William. *The Complete Poetry & Prose of William Blake.* Edited by David V. Erdman, Harold Bloom and William Golding. New York: Random House, 1988.

Blechschmidt, Erich. *The Ontogenetic Basis of Human Anatomy: A Biodynamic Approach to Development from Conception to Birth.* Edited and Translated by Brian Freeman. Berkeley: North Atlantic Books, 2004.

Boorstein, Seymour. *Transpersonal Psychotherapies.* Palo Alto, Calif.: Science and Behavior Books, 1980.

Boss, Medard. *A Psychiatrist Discovers India.* London: Wolff, 1965.

———. *Psychoanalysis and Daseinsanalysis.* Translated by Ludwig B. Lefebre. New York: Basic Books, 1963.

Briggs, George Weston. *Gorakhnath and the Kanphata Yogis.* Delhi: Motilal Banarsidass, 1982.

Broad, William. *The Science of Yoga: The Risks and the Rewards.* New York: Simon & Schuster, 2012.

Brooks, Douglas, Swami Durgananda, Paul Muller-Ortega, William Mahoney, Constantina Rhodes-Bailly, and S. P. Sabharathnam. *Meditation Revolution: A History and Theology of the Siddha Yoga Lineage.* South Fallsburg, N.Y.: Agama Press, 1997.

Brown, Gabrielle. *The New Celibacy.* New York: Ballantine, 1980.

Brown, Norman O. *Love's Body.* New York: Vintage, 1966.

Bubba Free John [Adi Da]. *Love of the Two-Armed Form.* Middletown, Calif.: Dawn Horse, 1978.

Buber, Martin. *I and Thou.* Translated by Ronald Gregor Smith. New York: Scribner's, 1958.

Bucknell, Roderick S., and Martin Stuart-Fox. *The Twilight Language: Explorations in Buddhist Meditation and Symbolism.* London: Curzon Press, 1986.

Buddhananda with Satyananda. *Moola Bandha: The Master Key.* Monghr, India: Goenka Bihar School of Yoga, 1978.

Campbell, Joseph. *The Power of Myth with Bill Moyers.* Edited by Betty Sue Flowers. New York: Doubleday, 1988.

Cantin, Marc, and Jacques Genest. "The Heart as an Endocrine Gland." *Clinical and Investigative Medicine* 9, no. 4 (1986): 319–27.

Carrellas, Barbara. *Urban Tantra: Sacred Sex for the Twenty-First Century.* Berkeley, Calif.: Celestial Arts, 2007.

Chamberlain, David B. *Consciousness at Birth: A Review of the Empirical Evidence.* San Diego: Chamberlain, 1983.

———. *The Mind of Your Newborn Baby.* 3rd ed. Berkeley, Calif.: North Atlantic Books, 1998.

Chesser, Eustace. *Salvation through Sex: The Life and Work of Wilhelm Reich.* New York: W. Morrow, 1973.

Chia, Mantak. *Taoist Secrets of Love: Cultivating Male Sexual Energy.* New York: Aurora, 1984.

Chia, Mantak, and Maneewan Chia. *Healing Love through the Tao: Cultivating Female Sexual Energy.* Rochester, Vt.: Destiny Books, 2005.

Clark, Keith. *Experience of Celibacy.* Notre Dame, Ind.: Ave Maria, 1982.

Clark, Ronald William. *Freud, the Man and the Cause.* London: J. Cape and Weidenfeld & Nicolson, 1980.

Cole, F. J. *Early Theories of Sexual Generation.* London: Oxford University Press, 1930.

Collins, Charles Dillard. *The Iconography and Ritual of Siva at Elephanta.* Albany: State University of New York Press, 1988.

Copernicus, Nicolaus. "Dedication of the Revolutions of the Heavenly Bodies to Pope Paul III." In *Harvard Classics, Famous Prefaces.* Edited by Charles W. Eliot. New York: P. F. Collier, 1969.

Courtright, Paul B. *Gaṇeśa: Lord of Obstacles, Lord of Beginnings.* New York: Oxford University Press, 1985.

Cowan, Connell, and Melvyn Kinder. *Smart Women, Foolish Choices.* New York: Random House, 1987.

Crews, Frederick C. "The Unknown Freud." In *The New York Review of Books* 40, no. 19 (November 18, 1993).

Curtis, Adam. *The Century of the Self.* British Broadcasting Co., 2002. Available at www.veoh.com/watch/v331913aKp43GXW (accessed February 6, 2014).

Dalrymple, William. *Nine Lives: In Search of the Sacred in Modern India.* London: Bloomsbury, 2009.

Daniélou, Alain. *The Complete Kama Sutra: The First Unabridged Modern Translation of the Classic Indian Text.* Rochester, Vt.: Inner Traditions, 1993.

Dass, Baba Hari. *Ashtanga Yoga Primer.* Santa Cruz, Calif.: Sri Rama, 1981.

———. *Hariakhan Baba: Known, Unknown.* Santa Cruz, Calif.: Sri Rama, 1975.

———. *Silence Speaks.* Santa Cruz, Calif.: Sri Rama, 1977.

———. *Sweeper to Saint: Stories of Holy India.* Santa Cruz, Calif.: Sri Rama, 1980.

Dass, Ram. *Remember, Be Here Now.* Cristobal, N. Mex.: Lama Foundation, 1971.

Dass, Ravi, and Aparna, eds. *The Marriage and Family Book: A Spiritual Guide.* New York: Schocken, 1978.

Davidson, Sara. "Ram Dass Has a Son! But Has This Revelation Changed His Conception of Love?" *Huffington Post,* November 3, 2010. www.huffingtonpost.com/sara-davidson/ram-dass-has-a-son_b_777452.html.

Deida, David. *The Enlightened Sex Manual: Sexual Skills for the Superior Lover.* Louisville, Colo.: Sounds True, 2007.

———. *Finding God through Sex: Awakening the One of Spirit through the Two of Flesh.* Boulder, Colo.: Sounds True, 2005.

———. *Naked Buddhism: 39 Ways to Free Your Heart and Awaken to Now.* Medford, N.J.: Plexus, 2002.

Delora, Joann S., and Carol A. B. Warren. *Understanding Sexual Interaction.* Boston: Houghton Mifflin, 1977.

DeMaria, Richard. *Communal Love at Oneida.* New York: Edwin Mellen, 1978.

D'Emilio, John, and Estelle B. Freedman. *Intimate Matters: A History of Sexuality in America.* New York: Harper & Row, 1988.

Demme, Jonathan. *Jimmy Carter: Man from Plains.* New York: Sony Pictures Classics, 2007.

de Nicolás, Antonio T. *Avatara: The Humanization of Philosophy Through the Bhagvad Gita.* New York: Nicolas Hays, 1976.

———, trans. *St. John of the Cross: Alchemist of the Soul.* New York: Paragon House, 1989.

de Ropp, Robert S. *Sex Energy.* New York: Delta, 1969.

de Rougemont, Denis. *Love in the Western World.* Translated by Montgomery Belgion. New York: Schocken, 1983.

Derrida, Jacques. *"Différance," Margins of Philosophy.* Chicago: University of Chicago Press, 1982.

Desai, Amrit. *Kripalu Yoga.* Lenox, Mass.: Kripalu Yoga Fellowship, 1985.

Dimock, Edward C. *The Place of the Hidden Moon.* Chicago: University of Chicago Press, 1966.

Dnyaneshwari Once Again. Translated by Swami Radhikananda Saraswati. Pune, India: Swami Radhikanand, 2002.

Donkin, William. *The Wayfarers: Meher Baba with the God-Intoxicated.* 1948. Hyderabad, India: Meher Mownavani Publications, 2002.

Douglas, Nik, and Penny Slinger. *Sexual Secrets.* Rochester, Vt.: Destiny Books, 1979.

Dychtwald, Ken. "Sexuality and the Whole Person." *Journal of Humanistic Psychology* 19, no. 2 (1979): 47–62.

Dyczkowski, Mark S. G., trans. *The Stanzas on Vibration.* Albany: State University of New York Press, 1992.

Eckhart, Meister. *Meister Eckhart: A Modern Translation.* Translated by Raymond B. Blakney. New York: Harper & Row, 1941.

Eisler, Riane. *The Chalice and the Blade.* New York: Harper & Row, 1987.

Eliade, Mircea. *Patanjali and Yoga.* New York: Schocken, 1976.

———. *Yoga: Immortality and Freedom.* Translated by William R. Trask. Princeton, N.J.: Princeton University Press, 1969.

Elizarenkova, Tatyana J. *Language and Style of the Vedic Rsis.* Albany: State University of New York Press, 1995.

Ellis, Havelock. *Psychology of Love.* New York: Mentor, 1933.

Evans-Wentz, W. Y. *The Tibetan Book of the Dead.* 1927. London: Oxford University Press, 1978.

Evola, Julius. *The Metaphysics of Sex.* Rochester, Vt.: Inner Traditions, 1983.

Feuerstein, Georg. *Encyclopedic Dictionary of Yoga.* New York: Paragon, 1990.

———. *Enlightened Sexuality.* Freedom, Calif.: Crossing Press, 1989.

———. *Textbook of Yoga.* London: Rider, 1975.

———. *Yoga: The Technology of Ecstasy.* Los Angeles: Jeremy P. Tarcher, 1989.

———. *The Yoga Tradition.* Prescott, Ariz.: Hohm Press, 1998.

———. *The Yoga-Sutra of Patanjali: A New Translation and Commentary.* Rochester, Vt.: Inner Traditions, 1990.

Fields, Rick. *How the Swans Came to the Lake: A Narrative History of Buddhism in America.* Boston: Shambhala, 1992.

Flood, Gavin. *The Tantric Body: The Secret Tradition of Hindu Religion.* London: I. B. Tauris, 2005.

Foucault, Michel. *Herculine Barbin: Being the Recently Discovered Memoirs of a Nineteenth-Century French Hermaphrodite.* Translated by Richard McDougall. New York: Pantheon, 1980.

———. *The History of Sexuality.* Translated by Robert Hurley. 3 vols. New York: Vintage, 1990.

———. *Technologies of the Self.* Edited by Luther H. Martin, et al. Amherst, Mass.: University of Massachusetts Press, 1988.

Fracchia, Charles A. *Living Alone Together: The New American Monasticism.* San Francisco: Harper & Row, 1979.

Freud, Sigmund. "Beyond the Pleasure Principle." 1920. In *The Freud Reader.* Edited by Peter Gay. New York: W. W. Norton, 1989.

———. *Civilization and its Discontents.* 1930. Translated by James Strachey. New York: Norton, 1961.

———. *The Future of an Illusion.* 1927. Translated by W. Robson-Scott. Garden City, N.Y.: Doubleday, 1961.

———. *The History of the Psychoanalytic Movement.* 1914. In *Basic Writings of Sigmund Freud.* Edited by A. A. Brill. New York: Modern Library, 1977.

———. *Sexuality and the Psychology of Love.* Edited by Philip Reiff. New York: MacMillan, 1963.

———. *Three Essays on the Theory of Sexuality.* 1905. Translated by James Strachey. New York: Avon, 1971.

Gilligan, Carol. *In a Different Voice: Psychological Theory and Women's Development.* Cambridge, Mass.: Harvard University Press, 1982.

Goldberg, Philip. *American Veda: From Emerson and the Beatles to Yoga and Meditation, How Indian Spirituality Changed the West.* New York: Random House, 2013.

Govindan, Marshall. *Babaji and the 18 Siddha Kriya Yoga Tradition.* 3rd ed. Montreal: Kriya Yoga Publications, 1993.

Gray, John. *Men Are from Mars, Women Are from Venus.* New York: HarperCollins, 1992.

Greer, Germaine. *Sex and Destiny.* New York: Harper & Row, 1984.

Gregoire, Carolyn. "What the F*ck Was Lululemon Thinking?" *Huffington Post,* October 22, 2013. www.huffingtonpost.com/carolyn-gregoire/what-the-fck-was-lululemon-thinking_b_4138754.html.

Guttmacher Institute. *Teenage Pregnancy: The Problem That Hasn't Gone Away.* New York: A. Guttmacher, 1981. More recent statistics available at www.guttmacher.org.

Haich, Elisabeth. *Sexual Energy and Yoga.* Translated by D. Stephenson. New York: Asi, 1972.

Haines, Richard Wheeler. *Handbook of Human Embryology.* Edinburgh: Churchill Livingston, 1972.

Harper, Katherine Anne, and Robert L. Brown, eds. *The Roots of Tantra.* Albany: State University of New York Press, 2002.

Hatcher, Robert A., et al. *Contraceptive Technology.* New York: Irvington, 1988.

Heidegger, Martin. *Being and Time.* 1927. Translated by John Macquarrie and Edward Robinson. New York: Harper & Row, 1962.

———. *Poetry, Language, Thought.* Translated by Albert Hofstadter. New York: Harper Colophon, 1975.

———. *What Is Called Thinking?* Translated by J. Glenn Gray. New York: Harper & Row, 1968.

Henderson, Julie. *The Lover Within: Opening to Energy in Sexual Practice.* Barrytown, N.Y.: Station Hill, 1987.

Hillman, James, and Michael Ventura. *We've Had a Hundred Years of Psychotherapy and the World's Getting Worse.* New York: HarperCollins, 1993.

Himes, Norman E. *Medical History of Contraception.* New York: Schocken, 1938.

Hite, Shere. *The Hite Report: A Nationwide Study of Female Sexuality.* New York: Dell, 1976.

———. *Women and Love: A Cultural Revolution in Progress.* New York: Knopf, 1987.

Huxley, Aldous. *Brave New World.* 1932. New York: Perennial, 1998.

Iyengar, B. K. S. *Light on Pranayama.* New York: Crossroad, 1981.

———. *Light on Yoga.* 1966. New York: Schocken, 1995.

Jnaneshvar, Shri. *Jnaneshvari.* Translated by V. G. Pradhan. Albany: State University of New York, 1987.

Johari, Harish. *Chakras: Energy Centers of Transformation.* Rochester, Vt.: Destiny Books, 1987.

Jones Payne Group, Inc. *Phase II Housing Needs Assessment and Demographic Analysis.* Window Rock, Ariz.: Navajo Housing Authority, 2008.

Kadloubovsky, E., and G. E. H. Palmer, trans. *Writings from the Philokalia, on Prayer of the Heart.* London: Faber, 1977.

Kagan, Jerome. *Unstable Ideas: Temperament, Cognition, and Self.* Cambridge, Mass.: Harvard University Press, 1989.

Kale, Arvind, and Shanta Kale. *Tantra: The Secret Power of Sex.* Bombay: Jaico, 1976.

Keleman, Stanley. *The Human Ground: Sexuality, Self and Survival.* Palo Alto, Calif.: Science and Behavior, 1975.

Kerr, Michael E., and Murray Bowen. *Family Evaluation.* New York: Norton, 1988.

Kierkegaard, Søren. *The Concept of Dread.* 1844. Translated by Walter Lowrie. Princeton, N.J.: Princeton University Press, 1973.

———. *The Present Age.* 1846. Translated by Alexander Dru. New York: Harper & Row, 1962.

———. *Works on Love.* 1847. Translated by Howard V. Hong and Edna H. Hong. New York: Harper Torchbook, 1962.

Kinsey, Alfred C., Wardell B. Pomeroy, and Clyde E. Martin. *Sexual Behavior in the Human Male.* Philadelphia: W. B. Saunders, 1948.

Kinsey, Alfred C., Wardell B. Pomeroy, Clyde E. Martin, and Paul H. Gebhard. *Sexual Behavior in the Human Female.* Philadelphia: W. B. Saunders, 1973.

Klein, Marty. *Sexual Intelligence: What We Really Want from Sex—and How to Get It*. New York: Harper Collins, 2012.

Koestenbaum, Peter. *Existential Sexuality*. Englewood Cliffs, N.J.: Prentice-Hall, 1974.

Kohn, Livia, and Robin R. Wang, eds. *Internal Alchemy*. Magdalena, N. Mex.: Three Pines Press, 2009.

Kohut, Heinz. *The Restoration of the Self*. New York: International Universities Press, 1977.

Kripalvananda. *Guru Prasad*. Summit Station, Pa.: Kripalu Yoga Fellowship, 1982.

———. *Pilgrimage of Love*. Vol. 3. Lenox, Mass.: Kripalu Yoga Fellowship, 1984.

———. *Revealing the Secret: A Commentary on the Small Burning Lamp of Sun-Moon Yoga (Hatha Yoga Pradipika)*. Edited by Charles Berner. Available at www.naturalmeditation.net/Design/meditation1RS.html.

———. *Science of Meditation*. Kayavarohan, India: D. H. Patel, 1977.

———. "Success or Freedom?" *Vishvamitra* 4, no. 1 (January 1977): 1–3.

Krishna, Gopi. *Kundalini: Path to Higher Consciousness*. New Delhi: Orient Paperbacks, 1992.

———. *Kundalini: The Evolutionary Energy in Man*. Berkeley: Shambhala, 1971.

Kuhn, Thomas S. *The Structure of Scientific Revolutions*. 1966. Chicago: University of Chicago Press, 1996.

Ladas, Alice Khan, Beverly Whipple, and John D. Perry. *The G Spot and Other Recent Discoveries about Human Sexuality*. 1982. New York: Holt, 2004.

Laing, R. D. *The Facts of Life*. London: Penguin, 1976.

———. *Knots*. New York: Pantheon, 1970.

———. *The Voice of Experience: Experience, Science and Psychiatry*. Harmondsworth, U. K. : Penguin, 1982.

Lao-tzu. *The Tao Te Ching: The Texts of Taoism*. Translated by James Legge. New York: Dover, 1962.

Lasch, Christopher. *The Culture of Narcissism: American Life in an Age of Diminishing Expectations*. Rev. ed. New York: W. W. Norton & Company, 1991.

Lati, Rinpoche, and Jeffrey Hopkins. *Death, Intermediate State and Rebirth in Tibetan Buddhism.* Valois, N.Y.: Gabriel/Snow Lion, 1981.

Lawrence, D. H. *The Plumed Serpent.* 1926. Edited by L. D. Clark. Cambridge: Cambridge University Press, 1987.

Lee, Chwen A., and Thomas G. Hand. *A Taste of Water: Christianity through Taoist-Buddhist Eyes.* New York: Pantheon, 1982.

Leonard, George. *The End of Sex.* Los Angeles: Jeremy P. Tarcher, 1983.

Liebowitz, Michael. *The Chemistry of Love.* Boston: Little, Brown, 1983.

Liu, Xun. "Numinous Father and Holy Mother: Late Ming Duo-Cultivation Practice." In *Internal Alchemy: Self, Society, and the Quest for Immortality,* edited by Livia Kohn and Robin R. Wang, 121–40. Magdalena, N.M.: Three Pines Press, 2009.

Longfellow, Henry Wadsworth. "The Ladder of Saint Augustine." 1858. www.poetryfoundation.org/poem/173902 (accessed December 23, 2013).

Lowen, Alexander. *Love and Orgasm.* New York: New American Library, 1967.

Luker, Kristin. *Taking Chances.* Berkeley: University of California Press, 1975.

Lukoff, D., F. Lu, and R. Turner. "Toward a More Culturally Sensitive DSM-IV. Psychoreligious and Psychospiritual Problems" In *Journal of Nervous and Mental Diseases* 180, no. 11 (1992): 673–82.

Ma, Shri Anandi. *This House Is on Fire: The Life of Shri Dhyanyogi.* Antioch, Calif.: Dhyanyoga Centers, 2005.

Maharaj, Nisargadatta. *I Am That.* Translated by Maurice Frydman. Bombay: Chetana, 1979.

Marcuse, Herbert. *Eros and Civilization.* 1955. Boston: Beacon, 1974.

Masters, William, Virginia E. Johnson, and Robert Kolodny. *Masters and Johnson on Sex and Human Loving.* Boston: Little, Brown, 1985.

McClelland, David C., and Carol Kirshnit. "The Effect of Motivational Arousal through Films on Salivary Immunoglobulin A." *Psychology and Health* 2, no. 1 (1988): 31–52.

McEvilley, Thomas. *The Shape of Ancient Thought: Comparative Studies in Greek and Indian Philosophies.* New York: Skyhorse Publishing, 2001. (See also http://buddhistartnews.wordpress.com/2013/08/23/12327. Accessed December 23, 2013.)

———. "The Spinal Serpent." In *The Roots of Tantra*. Edited by Katherine Anne Harper and Robert L. Brown. Albany: State University of New York Press, 2002.

McNeill, William H. *Keeping Together in Time*. Cambridge, Mass.: Harvard University Press, 1997.

Menzies, William W., and Robert P. Menzies. *Spirit and Power: Foundations of Pentecostal Experience*. Grand Rapids, Mich.: Zondervan, 2000.

Miller, Warren B., and Lucile F. Newman, eds. *The First Child and Family Formation*. Chapel Hill, N.C.: Carolina Population Center, University of North Carolina, 1978.

Millet, Kate. *Sexual Politics*. 1969. Garden City, N.Y.: Doubleday, 2000.

Money, John. *Love and Love Sickness*. Baltimore: Johns Hopkins University Press, 1980.

Montagu, Ashley. *Sex, Man and Society*. New York: Putnam, 1969.

Mookerjee, Ajit. *The Tantric Way*. Boston: Little, Brown, 1977.

Motoyama, Hiroshi. *Theories of the Chakras: Bridge to Higher Consciousness*. 1981. Wheaton, Ill.: Quest, 2008.

Muni, Rajarshi. *Yoga Experiences*. Kayavarohan, India: Patel, 1977.

Narayan, S. A. *The Beloved: A Song of Eternal Love*. Victoria, B.C.: Friesen Press, 2014.

Neill, Alexander Sutherland. *Summerhill: A Radical Approach to Child Rearing*. New York: Hart, 1960.

Nietzsche, Friedrich. *Thus Spake Zarathustra*. Translated by Walter Kaufmann. In *The Portable Nietzsche*. New York: Viking, 1970.

Nilsson, Lennart. Embryological photography. www.lennartnilsson.com (accessed December 23, 2013).

Oaklander, Nathan. "Sartre on Sex." In *The Philosophy of Sex*. Edited by Alan Soble. Totowa, N.J.: Littlefield, Adams, 1980.

Osho. *From Sex to Super-Consciousness*. 5th ed. India: Rebel Publishing House, 1996.

Pert, Candace B. *Molecules of Emotion: The Science Between Mind-Body Medicine*. New York: Scribner, 1999.

Pert, Candace B., and Nancy Marriott. *Everything You Need to Know to Feel Go(o)d*. Carlsbad, Calif.: Hay House, 2006.

Phelan, Nancy, and Michael Volin. *Sex and Yoga*. New York: Harper & Row, 1967.

Plato. *Timaeus*. 360 BCE. Translated by Benjamin Jowett. Available at http://classics.mit.edu/Plato/timaeus.html (accessed March 3, 2014).

Prabhavananda, Swami, and Christopher Isherwood. *How to Know God: Yoga Aphorisms of Patanjali*. New York: Signet, 1969.

Preller, Victor. *Divine Science and the Science of God: A Reformulation of Thomas Aquinas*. Princeton: Princeton University Press, 1967.

Prendergast, John, Peter Fenner, and Sheila Krystal, eds. *The Sacred Mirror: Nondual Wisdom and Psychotherapy*. St. Paul, Minn.: Paragon House, 2003.

Quine, W. V. *Ontological Relativity and Other Essays*. New York: Columbia University Press, 1969.

Radha, Swami Sivananda. *Kundalini: Yoga for the West*. Spokane, Wash.: Timeless Books, 1978.

Rama, Swami, Rudolphy Ballantine, and Swami Ajaya. *Yoga and Psychotherapy: The Evolution of Consciousness*. Honesdale, Pa.: Himalayan Institute, 1979.

Ramakrishnan, K. K., ed. *Who Is Meher Baba?* Poona, India: Meher Era, 1995.

Ramanujan, A. K., ed. and trans. *Speaking of Siva*. Baltimore: Penguin, 1973.

Ramaswamy, Krishnan, Antonio de Nicolas, and Aditi Banerjee. *Invading the Sacred: An Analysis of Hinduism Studies in America*. New Delhi: Rupa & Co., 2007.

Raphael, Sally J. *Finding Love*. New York: Jove, 1984.

Rawson, Philip. *The Indian Cult of Ecstasy: Tantra*. New York: Bounty, 1973.

Ray, Satyajit. *Pather Panchali* [Song of the Little Road]. India: Government of West Bengal; Aurora Film Co., 1955.

Reich, Wilhelm. *The Function of the Orgasm*. Translated by Vincent R. Carfagano. New York: Simon & Schuster, 1973.

———. *The Sexual Revolution*. Translated by Theodore P. Wolfe. New York: Farrar, Strauss, and Giroux, 1974.

Reik, Theodor. *The Psychology of Sex Relations*. New York: Farrar & Reinhart, 1948.

Rein, G., and R. M. McCraty. "Long-Term Effects of Compassion on Salivary IgA." *Psychosomatic Medicine* 56, no. 2 (1994): 171–72.

Rein, Glen, Mike Atkinson, and Rollin McCraty. "The Physiological and Psychological Effects of Compassion and Anger." *Journal of Advancement in Medicine* 8, no. 2 (1995): 87–105.

Richardson, Diana. *The Heart of Tantric Sex: A Unique Guide to Love and Sexual Fulfillment*. Hants, UK: Mantra Books, 2003.

Rieker, Hans-Ulrich. *The Yoga of Light*. Translated by Elys Becherer. Los Angeles: Dawn Horse Press, 1971.

Rig Veda. Translated by Ralph T. H. Griffith. Available at www.sanskritweb .net/rigveda/griffith.pdf.

Roszak, Theodore. *The Making of a Counter Culture*. Garden City, N.Y.: Anchor, 1969.

Russianoff, Penelope. *Why Do I Think I Am Nothing Without a Man?* New York: Bantam, 1983.

Ryan, Christopher, and Cacilda Jethá. *Sex at Dawn: How We Mate, Why We Stray, and What It Means for Modern Relationships*. New York: Harper Perennial, 2011.

Saint John of the Cross. *The Dark Night of the Soul*. Translated by Kurt F. Reinhardt. New York: Ungar, 1957.

Saint-Exupéry, Antoine de. *The Little Prince*. 1943. Translated by Katherine Woods. New York: Harvest/Harcourt Brace Jovanovich, 1971.

Salzberg, Sharon, and Robert Thurman. *Love Your Enemies: How to Break the Anger Habit & Be a Whole Lot Happier*. New York: Hay House, 2013.

Samuel, Geoffrey. *The Origins of Yoga and Tantra: Indic Religions to the Thirteenth Century*. New York: Cambridge University Press, 2008.

Sannella, Lee. *The Kundalini Experience*. Lower Lake, Calif.: Integral Press, 1987. (First published in 1977 under the title *Kundalini: Psychosis or Transcendence?*)

Sarbacker, Stuart Ray. "Herbs (*auṣadhi*) as a Means to Spiritual Accomplishments (*siddhi*) in Patañjali's *Yogasūtra*." *International Journal of Hindu Studies* 17, no. 1 (April 2013): 37–56.

Sartre, Jean Paul. *Being and Nothingness: An Essay on Phenomenological Ontology*. Translated by Hazel Barnes. New York: Philosophical Library, 1956.

Satyeswarananda, Giri. *Babaji: The Divine Himalayan Yogi*. Vol 1. San Diego, Calif.: Sanskrit Classics, 1993.

Schurmann, Reiner. *Heidegger on Being and Acting: From Principles to Anarchy*. Translated by Christine-Marie Gros. Bloomington: Indiana University Press, 1987.

Scruton, Roger. *Sexual Desire: A Moral Philosophy of the Erotic*. New York: Free Press, 1986.

Silburn, Lilian. *Kundalini: The Energy of the Depths.* Translated by Jacques Gontier. Albany: State University of New York Press, 1988.

Singer, June. *Androgyny: Toward a New Theory of Sexuality.* Garden City, N.Y.: Anchor Doubleday, 1977.

Singleton, Mark. *Yoga Body: The Origins of Modern Posture Practice.* New York: Oxford University Press, 2010.

Shaw, Eric. "The Timeless Tradition of Naked Yoga." *Common Ground Magazine,* January 2010.

Singh, Lalan Prasad. *Tantra: Its Mystic and Scientific Basis.* Delhi: Concept Publishing, 1976.

Sivananda. *Kundalini Yoga.* Sivanandanagar, India: Divine Light, 1971.

Sjoman, N. E. *The Yoga Tradition of the Mysore Palace.* New Delhi: Abhinav Publications, 1999.

Smith, Frederick M. *The Self Possessed: Deity and Spirit Possession in South Asian Literature and Civilization.* New York: Columbia University Press, 2006.

Sovatsky, Stuart. "Clinical Contemplations on Impermanence: Temporal and Linguistic Factors in Client Hopelessness." *Review of Existential Psychology and Psychiatry* 21, nos. 1–3 (1993): 153–79.

———. "Clinical Forms of Love Inspired by Meher Baba's Mast Work." *Journal of Transpersonal Psychology* 36, no. 2 (2004): 134–49.

———. "Divine Mothering Separation Anxiety." In *Facets of Consciousness.* Edited by T. V. Gopal. SCSVM, Tamil, Nadu, India, 2007.

———. "Eros as Mystery: The Shared-Gender Mystery." *Journal of Humanistic Psychology* 33, no. 2 (Spring 1993): 72–90.

———. "Eros as Mystery: Toward a Transpersonal Sexology and Procreativity." *Journal of Transpersonal Psychology* 17, no. 1 (1985): 1–32.

———. "Euro-Hinduism in America: From Vivekananda to Deepak Chopra." In *Columbia Desk Reference on Eastern Religions.* Edited by Robert Thurman. Contracted by Columbia University Press. Tabled, 2002. Available at http://merliannews.com/Yoga_35/Euro-Hinduism_in_America_From_Vivekananda_to_Deepak_Chopra_by_Stuart_Sovatsky_Part_One_printer.shtml.

———. "From Foucault's Ars Erotica to the Next Wave of Inwardly Inspired Yoga and 'Tantric Sex.'" In *Journal of Holistic Psychology 2* (2013), chapter 12.

———. "Kundalini and the Complete Maturation of the Ensouled Body." *Journal of Transpersonal Psychology* 41, no. 1 (2009): 1–21.

———. "Kundalini: Breakthrough or Breakdown?" *Yoga Journal* 63 (July 1985): 42–43.

———. *Love Secrets* [in Russian]. Edited by A. Rye. Moscow: Amaria Rye, 2012.

———. "Meher Baba and Psychotherapy of Love." In *Psychology of Health and Well-Being: Some Emerging Issues.* Edited by Sandhya Ojha. Varanasi, India, 2009.

———. "On Being Moved: Kundalini and the Complete Maturation of the Ensouled Body." In *Internal Alchemy.* Edited by Livia Kohn and Robin R. Wang. Magdalena, N. Mex.: Three Pines Press, 2009.

———. *A Phenomenological Exploration of Orgasmic, Tantric and Brahmacharya Sexualities.* Ann Arbor, Mich.: University Microfilms, 1984.

———. "The Pleasures of Celibacy." *Yoga Journal* (March 1987).

———. "Project Together: A Comprehensive-Preventative Approach to School Incorrigibility and Minor Delinquent Behavior." Atlantic County Youth Services (S. L. E. P. A. Grant A-178-75), 1977.

———. "Psychopathology and DSM-IV Religious Issues." *Review of Existential Psychiatry and Psychology* 25, nos. 1–3 (2001): 93–103.

———. "Ram Dass Has a Son! . . . and then he began to see." *Association for Humanistic Psychology Newsletter* (May 2012).

———. Review of *Integral Psychology: Yoga, Growth and Opening the Heart.* *Journal of Transpersonal Psychology* 43, no. 1 (2011). Available at http://atpweb.org/jtparchive/trps-43-11-01-104.pdf.

———. "Spiritual Depths of Admiration in Family Therapy: Grihastha: Family Life as a Spiritual Path." In *Consciousness, Indian Psychology and Yoga.* Edited by K. Joshi and M. Cornellisen. Delhi, India: Centre for Studies in Civilization, 2004.

———. "Spirituality and Psychotherapy: The Matter of 'Separation Anxiety' and Beyond." *International Journal of Transpersonal Studies* 20 (2001): 79–84.

———. "Stuart Sovatsky on Partner Yoga and Tantra Yoga" [in Russian] *Yoga Journal Russia* (February 2009): 74–79.

———. "Tantric Celibacy and Erotic Mystery." In *Enlightened Sexuality.*

Edited by Georg Feuerstein. Freedom, Calif.: Crossing Press, 1989.

———. *Words from the Soul: Time, East/West Spirituality and Psychotherapeutic Narrative.* Albany: State University of New York Press, 1998.

———. *Your Perfect Lips.* Lincoln, Neb.: iUniverse, 2005.

Spinoza, Benedict de. *Works of Spinoza.* Translated by R. H. M. Elwes. New York: Dover, 1951.

Stanford Encyclopedia of Philosophy. "Descartes and the Pineal Gland." http://plato.stanford.eduentries/pineal-gland (accessed December 30, 2012).

Steinhoff, P. "Premarital Pregnancy and the First Birth." In *The First Child and Family Formation.* Edited by Warren B. Miller and Lucile F. Newman. Chapel Hill: Carolina Population Center, University of North Carolina, 1978.

Stern, Daniel N. *The Interpersonal World of the Infant.* New York: Basic, 1985.

Suranna, Pingali. *The Demon's Daughter, A Love Story from South India.* Translated by Velcheru Narayana Rao and David Shulman. Albany: State University of New York Press, 2006.

Svoboda, Robert E. *Aghora, At the Left Hand of God.* Albuquerque, N. Mex.: Brotherhood of Life, 1986.

Syman, Stefanie. *The Subtle Body: The Story of Yoga in America.* New York: Farrar, Straus and Giroux, 2011.

Symons, Donald. *The Evolution of Human Sexuality.* Santa Barbara, Calif.: University of Santa Barbara Press, 1979.

Szasz, Thomas. *Sex by Prescription: The Startling Truth about Today's Sex Therapy.* Garden City, NY: Anchor, 1980.

Taimini, I. K. *The Science of Yoga.* Wheaton, Ill.: Quest, 1967.

Tart, Charles T., ed. *Transpersonal Psychologies.* New York: Harper Colophon, 1975.

The Secret of the Golden Flower. Available at http://thesecretofthegolden flower.com (accessed December 23, 2013).

Thirumoolar. *Thirumandiram: A Classic of Yoga and Tantra, Vols. 1–3.* Edited by Marshall Govindan. Translated by B. Natarajan. Montreal: Kriya Yoga, 1993.

Thurman, Robert. *Inner Revolution: Life, Liberty, and the Pursuit of Real Happiness.* New York: Penguin, 1999.

Tolle, Eckhart. *A New Earth: Awakening to Your Life's Purpose*. New York: Dutton, 2005.

———. *The Power of Now: A Guide to Spiritual Enlightenment*. New York: New World Library, 2004.

Tripp, C. A. *The Homosexual Matrix*. New York: McGraw-Hill, 1975.

Tweed, Thomas A., and Stephen Prothero. *Asian Religions in America*. New York: Oxford University Press, 1999.

Urban, Hugh B. *Tantra: Sex, Secrecy, Politics, and Power in the Study of Religions*. Berkeley: University of California Press, 2003.

Van Kaam, Adrian L. "Sex and Existence." In *Readings in Existential Phenomenology*. Edited by Nathaniel Morris Lawrence and Daniel Denis O'Connor. Englewood Cliffs, N.J.: Prentice-Hall, 1967.

Vasu, Rai Bahadur Srisa Chandra, trans. *The Siva Samhita*. New Delhi: Oriental Book Reprint Co., n.d.

Venkatesananda, Swami. *The Concise Yoga Vasistha*. Albany: State University of New York Press, 1984.

Verny, Thomas, with John Kelly. *The Secret Life of the Unborn Child*. New York: Dell, 1981.

Vishnu Tirtha. *Devatma Shakti (Kundalini): Divine Power*. Rishikesh, India: Vigyan Press, 1993.

Vishnu-devananda, Swami. *The Complete Illustrated Book of Yoga*. 1960. New York: Harmony, 1995.

Vissell, Barry, and Joyce Vissell. *The Shared Heart*. Aptos, Calif.: Ramira, 1984.

Vyas Dev Ji, Swami. *Science of Soul*. Rishikesh, India: Yoga Niketan Trust, 1972.

Wallerstein, Judith S., Julia M. Lewis, and Sandra Blakeslee. *The Unexpected Legacy of Divorce: The 25 Year Landmark Study*. New York: Hyperion, 2001.

Wallis, Christopher D. *Tantra Illuminated*. The Woodlands, Tex.: Anusara Press, 2012.

Washburn, Michael. *The Ego and the Dynamic Ground: A Transpersonal Theory of Human Development*. Albany: State University of New York Press, 1995.

Webster, Richard. *Why Freud Was Wrong: Sin, Science, and Psychoanalysis*. New York: Basic Books, 1995.

Wedemeyer, Christian K. *Making Sense of Tantric Buddhism: History, Semiology, and Transgression in the Indian Traditions.* New York: Columbia University Press, 2012.

Welwood, John. *Journey of the Heart.* New York: Harper Collins, 1990.

Whitaker, Carl A., and William M. Bumberry. *Dancing with the Family: A Symbolic-Experiential Approach.* New York: Routledge, 1988.

White, David Gordon. *The Alchemical Body.* Chicago: University of Chicago Press, 1996.

———. *Kiss of the Yogini, "Tantric Sex" in Its South Asian Contexts.* Chicago: University of Chicago Press, 2003.

———. *Sinister Yogis.* Chicago: University of Chicago Press, 2009.

———, ed. *Tantra in Practice.* Princeton, N.J.: Princeton University Press, 2000.

White, Michael. *Narrative Practice: Continuing the Conversations.* New York: W. W. Norton, 2011.

Wilber, Ken. "Are the Chakras Real?" In *Kundalini, Evolution and Enlightenment.* Edited by John White. Garden City, N.Y.: Anchor, 1979.

———. *Sex, Ecology, Spirituality: The Spirit of Evolution.* 1995. Boston: Shambhala, 2001.

———. *Up From Eden.* Garden City, N.Y.: Anchor Doubleday, 1981.

Wittgenstein, Ludwig. *On Certainty.* Edited by G. E. M. Anscombe and G. H. von Wright. Translated by Denis Paul and G. E. M. Anscombe. New York: Harper, 1969.

———. *Philosophical Investigations: The English Text of the Third Edition.* Translated by G. E. M. Anscombe. New York: Macmillan, 1968.

Woodroffe, Sir John. *Principles of Tantra.* 1914. Madras, India: Ganesh, 1978.

Yogananda, Paramahansa. *Autobiography of a Yogi.* 1946. Los Angeles: Self-Realization Fellowship, 1977.

Yu, Eunice, and Jianguo Liu. "Environmental Impacts of Divorce." Edited by Paul R. Ehrlich, Stanford University. *Proceedings of the National Academy of Sciences* 104, no. 5 (October 30, 2007): 20629–34.

Yu, Lu K'uan. *Taoist Yoga: Alchemy and Immortality.* York Beach, Me.: Samuel Weiser, 1973.

Zvelebil, Kamil V. *The Siddha Quest for Immortality.* New York: Red Wheel Weiser, 1996.

Index

Numbers in *italics* indicate illustrations.

abortion
  as contraceptive failure, 79, 133
  debate over, 38, 55, 79
  frustration with, 72, 79
abuse, 65–67, 120
  sexual, 55–56, 92
  social-political, 64
addictions, 4
advaita, 105
advertising, 8, 24
agnisara dhauti, 211
ahamkara, 89
Alternate Breathing, practice, 150
ambiguity, 32, *36*
  in emotions, 167, 172
  as erotic innuendoes, 39–41
  "too good to be true," 125
amrita, 26
  hypothalamus-pineal puberty,
    98–99
  khechari mudra and, 103
  orgasm and overconsumption
    debate, 102

apology, 67, 77, 87, 167–68, 193
ars erotica, 85–89
  of bhakti yoga, 95
  defined, 3
  future societies, 133
  partner yoga, 78
  scientia sexualis versus, *4, 5*
  shift from scientia sexualis, 25–30
  teenagers and, 145–49
  as yogic path, 8
  See also dancing; hatha yoga;
    Nyasa; uju kaya; sublimation
asana, as postures, 202–5
  spontaneous, *8–9, 17,* 73, 102,
    225–26
  as surrendered worship, 224
ascetic, 210
  naga yogi, 12
asvini mudra, 215
atman, 88. *See also* soul
attractions, 2, 22, 76, 145, 154
"awaiting the beloved," 224
Axis Mundi, 20, 185

bandhas (locks), 199–201
  spontaneously arising, 207, 247
bhakti, 69, 77, 118, 180, 198. *See
  also* ars erotica; lila; twilight
  teachings
Bhastrika, practice, 213
belly dancing, 9–10, 185, 223–24
"beyond the pale," 234–38
Bhadra-asana (Nobility Pose
  Tumescence), 205
Bhagavad-Gita, 103, 105
bliss body, 88–89
blushing, 43, 129, 163, 178
brahmacharya, 14, 71–75, 80–83
  147–148, 202
  early stages of, 175–76
  "gradual brahmacharya," 194–95
  for older couples, 247
  urdhvaretas, 26
  See also celibacy
Breathing Mystery, practice, 187
Broad, William, 25, 106
Brown, Gabrielle (*The New Celibacy*),
  74
Buber, Martin (*I and Thou*), 67, 175
Buddha, 11, 74, 249
  enlightenment of, 110
Buddhism, as a still-sitting meditative
  path, 9–10

celibacy, 6, 74, 80, 95, 190. *See also*
  brahmacharya
chakras, 42, 85, 90
  activation practice, 213
  ajna, 97–100
  anahata, 92–95

manipura, 91–92
  muladhara, 90–91
  sahasrara, 100–101
  svadhisthana, 91
  vishuddha, 95–97
chanting, 18, 73, 95–96, 187. *See also*
  kirtan; mantra
commitment, 120–21
  fear of, 120
  lifelong, 121
  as loyalty to mystery, 117–19
  to possibility, 78
  solitary brahmacharya and, 77
communication, 13, 118, 127
  meditation awareness and, 210
  negative patterns of, 168
  nonverbal, 167
  problem solving practices, 169–74
  See also dialogue
compassion, 10, 92–94, 98
conception, 2, 140, 143–44
contraception, 79, 80, 133
Cornucopia, practice, 216
couples, 47, 78, 100, 118
  childless, 70, 146, 236
  older couples, 247–48
  See also yoga
Crescent Moon, posture, 218
cyberpornography, 27. *See also*
  pornography
cynicism, 35–36, 42, 111, 156

dancing, 49, 65, 148, 185, 247
Dass, Baba Hari, 198, 210, 238–39,
  241, 245
Dass, Ram, 29, 88, 246

death, 66, 101, 110, 128, 146
demystification of eros, 59, 130
desire, 26, 69, 94, 185, 216
destiny, 143
devotion, 10, 58, 62, 109, 188
dharana, 107, 178–79, 187
    Christian version of, 109
dhyana, 107, 109–10, 179, 182
dialogue, transformation of, 156
diet, 16, 190–91
Divine Mother Kundalini, 72
divorce, 26, 116–17, 119, 122
    dating scene, 146
    rates of, 30, 117, 166
divya sharira, 11, 103
drugs, 148–49
    instant enlightenments, 16
Dual Yoga Mudra, Standing, 219

ecstasy, 99, 119, 148
ego-self, 89
embarrassment, 41, 47, 130
entheogenic rasas, 88, 137, 180, 195,
    197
envy, transmutation of, 130
eros, as mystery, 33, 51
erotic, 61–64. See also viyoga

faith, 42, 62–63, 77–78, 94, 111
family, 29, 122, 146, 169
    family practices, 215
fantasies, 34, 43–44, 71, 86, 91
fasting, 191
fertility, 64, 68–69, 102, 132–34,
    140–42
flirtation, 27, 55, 243

forgiveness, 77, 92, 193, 196
    shyness and, 129
Foucault, Michel, 2–3, 20, 27, 53,
    122
freedom of belonging, 130–31
Freud, Sigmund, limited views of, 5,
    7–8, 16, 78
friendship, nonsexual, 76

Gandhi, Mahatma, 19, 74, 87, 99, 147
gender, as over-differentiating, 52,
    55
    ecology of, 51–52, 58
    shared immersion in mystery,
        51–63
gestation, 90, 137, 140, 143
    relational worship practices during,
        144
    "return to the womb," 103
God/Goddess, 65, 96, 234, 241–42
grace, 93, 122, 159, 224
    as a practice, 215
Grand Yogaverse, 48
gratitude, 44, 78, 129, 163, 195
    shyness and, 76, 129
Great Gesture practice, 177, 187,
    190
grief, 4, 68, 76, 130, 144
grihastha, 8, 10, 29, 91, 123, 247. See
    also commitment; marriage
group practice, 183–84, 187–88
guru, 81, 100

Hala-asana (Plow Pose Tumescence),
    203
Hammarskjöld, Dag, 74

harassment, sexual, 56
hatha yoga, 198–210
  as ars erotica, 198–99
  as spontaneous movement, 224–25
  See also sahaja yoga
Hatha Yoga Pradipika, 244
heart, seeing with, 77
Hearts and Backs, practice, 217
hidden union, 127. *See also* viyoga
HIV, conflictual problems of, 75, 83
home-building, 69, 188
homophobia, 37, 55
  limiting of sexual freedom and,
    146
homosexuality, 37, 68
hospice practice, 214
humility, 60, 90, 130, 176, 241–42
humor, 55, 190, 192–93
hypothalamus, 98, 176, 202, 243,
  245

immortality, 34, 61, 101. *See also*
  mortality
impermanence, 43–44, 47
incest, 45
inner adult, 178, 183
inner child, 38
Inner Empathic Spaces (IES), 151,
  153–55, 235
inner marriage, 11, 19, 50, 105
innocence, diminished by
    judgmentalism, 124–25, 193
  as erotic contact, 146
intelligence, 85–86, 91, 109, 224
intercourse, 58, 106
  of anointing, 71 (*see also* Nyasa)

frequency, 102
  verbal, 167
intimacy, 44–45, 178–79
  deepening of, 76, 85–86
  fear of, 46
intimus, *36,* 48–49, 85, 118–19,
  156–57
I-Thou, 171, 175
Iyengar, B. K. S. (*Light on Yoga*),
  199

Jainism, as a still-sitting meditative
    path, 9
jalandhara bandha, 50, 200
jealousy, 91
  transmutation of, 130
jiva, 85, 88, 135–36. *See also* soul
Jnaneshvari-gita, 224
John of the Cross, Saint, 244
joy, 78, 86, 99, 105, 154
Judeo-Christian traditions, as still
    sitting meditative path, 9

kaivalya, 101, 107, 110
Kama Sutra, 14
kapala-bhati, 201, 225
karma, 74, 110, 247
karma yoga, 74
khechari mudra, 18, 26, 102–3
  as tumescence, 50
kirtan, 5, 20, 72, 84, 195. *See* also
    chanting; Axis Mundi
kiss, as lover's devotion, 236
  singular ars erotica, 185–86
  triggered by joy, 153
koan, 126

kosha (subtle body), 85–86
  ananda-maya, 23, 85–86, 88–89
  anna-maya, 85–86, 100–101
  mano-maya, 85–86
  prana-maya, 85–86, 224
  vijnana-maya, 87–88
Kripalvananda, Swami, 106, 207,
    225, 241, 244
  Lakulisha and, 246
Krishna, Gopi, 22–24, 90–91
kumbhaka, 200, 225
kundalini
  allured upward by ojas, 92
  awakening of, 10, 23–24, 145
  genius and, 91
Kurma Purana, 246

labeling, 41, 68, 172
Lakulisha, 246–47
language
  creating a world and, 68
  humor and, 190
  suggestiveness and, 33, 43, 176
  twilight language, 238
Lao-tzu (Tao Te Ching), 43, 190
Lawrence, D. H. (The Plumed
    Serpent), 34
"letting go," 70, 81, 247–48
lila, 12, 151
  in bhakti yoga, 118
Linga Purana, 246
longing, in bhakti yoga, 69
  in viyogic union, 127, 130
Lord Prana, 137. See also prana
love, anahata chakra, 92–94
  unbreakable, 10, 152, 170

  unconditional, 121, 151–52
  See also prema

Mahadeviyakka, 127
maha mudra, 200, 211
Malebranche, 111
mantra, 17, 42, 81, 108
  chanting practice, 187–88
  inner mantra meditation, 210
  See also pratyahara
Marcuse, Herbert, repressive
    de-sublimation 24
marriage, 26–30, 78, 121, 133, 146,
    151
Masters and Johnson and artificial
    wombs, 133
masturbation, 81, 102, 147
  opposing views of, 38
maturation, 20, 29, 93, 102–3
  lifelong, 42, 118, 197
  physical-spiritual, four types of,
    10–11
meditation, 62, 74, 105–9, 117, 213
  advanced practices, 210
  before yoga practices, 198
  during lovemaking, 195
Meditation for All, practice, 213
menopause, 188
midlife crisis, 247
missing another, 127–30, 152, 158
  sublimation and, 227
money, 4, 44, 121
Money, John, 106
monogamy, 121–22
  lifelong loyal, 122
  serial, 1, 30, 122

mortality, 100, 118
  known via impermanence, 44–45
  See also immortality
motivations for brahmacharya,
    83–84
  to deepen intimacy, 76
  desire for solitude, 75
  to develop nonsexual friendships,
    76
  to enhance marriage, 78
  frustration with contraception,
    79–80
  health, 75
  as problematic, 83
  support for creativity 74
  to transform relational struggles,
    77–78
mudras, 200–201, 211–12
  defined, 8
  meditative intimus as, 49
  spontaneous 102, 106
mystery, 44–48
  entering the aura of, *36*
  an essence of eros, 32–33
  gender as shared, 51–66
  of hidden potential, 119
  movement toward, 43
Mystery of Balance practice, 183–84,
    184

nabhan mudra, 201, 213
nadi shodhana sahita kumbhaka,
    202, 210
Nicephorus the Solitary, 109
nirbija-samadhi, 110
nonattachment, 76, 89, 97, 186

nondualism. See *advaita*
Not-Enough-Time Routine, practice,
    210
Nyasa, 71, 73, 141, *181,* 188
  empowerment of chakras, 182
  practice of, 180–82

ojas, 26, 92–94, 102
  as body constitutents, 101–2
  manipura chakra and, 91–92
One-Word Ritual, practice, 190
  as recovery word tool, 64–67
orgasm, 102, 107, 151, 185, 191, 195
"owning" sexuality, limitations of
  concept of, 64–67

Padma-asana (Lotus Pose
    Tumescence), 162, 205
pariyanga, 6–10, 26–27, 79, 232,
    235–36
Pashchimottana-asana (Seated Head-
    to-Knee, Back-Stretching Pose
    Tumescence), 204, 208–9
Patanjali (*Yoga Sutras*), 107
polyamory, 1, 4, 7, 71
  lifelong loyal, 122
pornography, 38. *See also*
  cyberpornography
power struggles, 4
Prabhu, Allama, 100
prana, 102, 224–25
  sub-pranas, 210, 225
  See also Lord Prana
pranayama, 201–2, 207, 210–11
  spontaneous, 225–26
Pranic Mirroring practice, 185

pranotthana, 102, 145. *See also* Divine Mother Kundalini

pratyahara, 107–8, 177, 180, 185–87

pregnancy, 144, 188
  unintended, 79
  See also relational worship practices

prema, 97, 110. *See also* love

prenatal yoga, 215

"pre-transpersonal fallacy," 92

procreation, 10, 79, 140–42
  mystery of, 13

Ramakrishna, 82

rasa, 48, 79, 98, 103

Reich, Wilhelm, 8, 25, 79

relational worship practices, 144, 148, 170

repression, 24, 38

respect, 54–55, 65–67, 87, 129

restricted-movement practice, 214

retas, 9, 13, 24–26, 75, 103, 120
  meditation, 134

Rilke, Rainer Maria (*Duino Elegies*), 66, 111

ritual worship, 108
  of mystery, 188

sabija-samadhi, 107, 110

sadhana
  as formal practice, 236
  as love partner, 75

safe sex, 73, 191

sahaja yoga, 102, 106, 143, 224, 227

Sannella, Lee, 5, 23

sannyasa, 247

Sara hasta bhujanga-asana (King Cobra Tumescence), 206, 209

Sarvanga-asana (shoulder stand), 204, 208–9

scientia sexualis, *4,* 12, 24–25, 76, 114
  shift from, 25–26

Secret Knowledge Ritual, practice, 190

secret teachings. *See* twilight teachings

seed, 57, 86, 101, 235
  potentials, 2, 9, 125
  See also retas

sensate focusing, 107

sex-desire, 25, 27, 68, 140, 194

sex education, 80
  reinterpreted via mystery, 145

sex therapy, 107

sexual images as metaphors, 94

sexually transmitted diseases, 75

shadow, 55

shaktipat, 17, 29, 33, 49, 244

shame, 47, 129–30, 194

shared-gender mystery, 51–55, 56–58, 65, 79, 143

Shirsa-asana (Headstand Tumescence), 204

Shiva-Shakti, 10, 33, 67, 189, 196

Siddha-asana (Adept Pose Tumescence), 139, 162, 206

Sikhism, as a still-sitting meditative path, 9

silence, 75, 109, 142, 167

singing, 55, 148, 246–47. *See also* chanting

skepticism, 35
sleep, 190–91
social media, 1, 8
solitary as practice, 198
    as spiritual life, 241
Song of Solomon, 180
soteriology, secret power in the word,
    67
soul, 47–48, 66–67, 85, 88, 92–94
Sovatsky Method Couples
    Counseling, 6
spinal puberties, 91, 106, 118, 195–97.
    See also Thirumandiram;
    twilight teachings
Spinoza, Baruch, 89
Sringara Rasa, 14, 91, 155, 235–38
    bliss and wonder of, 142
    "enlightenment realms," 234
    esoteric circles and, 234
    as long term state, 23
    poetic example, 228–31
sublimation, 9, 69, 227
    nuance of, 191
    reconciliation, 194
Sunrise Ritual, practice, 190
synchronicity, 178
systems theory, 57

tantra, 60, 90, 192
    neo-tantra, 11–12, 25–26, 29,
        32
    pariyanga, 8–9
    "tantric sex" as oxymoron, 12
tantric brahmacharya, 83, 175, 185,
    194
tears as erotic secretions, 178

teenagers, 8, 13, 80, 146–49
    Alternate Breathing practice, 150
    brahmacharya and, 80, 147–48
    relational worship practices, 148
    Yourself Breathing practice,
        149–50
Teresa, Mother, 74
Thirumandiram of Siddhar,
    Thirumoolar, 232–34
Thurman, Robert, 19
Tirtha, Swami Vishnu (Devatma
    Shakti), 198
trust, 37, 54, 60, 86, 145
tumescence, 2, 50, 67, 178–79, 199.
    See also khechari mudra
turning away, 46
twilight teachings, 105, 231–35,
    238–39
    in Khajuraho Temple carvings, 231
    in Tibetan tangka, 231
    See also "beyond the pale"; Sringara
        Rasa
Twin Boats practice, 221–22
Twin Cobras practice, 220
Twin Dancers' practice, 223
Twin Plows practice, 222

union, 77, 110, 127, 151
    in sacred art, 231, 232
uju kaya, 9–10
urdhvaretas, 70–72, 81, 92–93,
    168–69, 176
    defined 1–3, 17
    maturation of, 8
    matured conjugal, 65
    mystery, 35, 36

sexual orientation in, 148
"V" practice, 221
yoga, 10, 70, 75, 79–80
uvulas, 244–45

vairagha, 97. *See also* nonattachment
Vayu Purana, 246
verbal asanas of creative
    communication, 167–74
Verny, Thomas (*The Secret Life of the
    Unborn Child*), 143
vidya. *See* wisdom
vinyasa, 225
Viparita karani mudra (Reverse Pose
    Tumescence), 203
virya, 26, 94, 102, 178
viyoga, 77, 126–29, 164–65
vows, 75, 188, 191–93
vulnerability, 65, 108
Vyas Dev, 89, 100

White, David G. (*The Alchemical
    Body*), 246
Whitman, Walt (*Unseen Buds*), 132
Wilber, Ken, 92
wisdom, 97, 105, 119
    defined, 88–89
wonderment, 178
Woodroffe, John (Avalon, Arthur), 105

world family, 100, 119, 165, 235
worship, 118, 130, 180, 195–96
    endless erotic, 26
    gender worship, 61–63
    seed-rasa-mudra-activating, 63

xenophobia, 130

yama, 201
yoga
    ars erotica practices, 170
    boudoir yoga, 6, 22 (*see also*
        pariyanga*)
    chair and bed yoga, 214
    Christian Yoga, 72–73
    communication yoga, 151
    daily practice, 207–10
    marrying, 17
    nude yoga classes, 10
    partner yoga, 78, 215–23
    spontaneous, 242
    video yoga course, 215
    See also sahaja yoga
yoga mudra, 206, 208–9. *See also*
    Dual Yoga Mudra, Standing
Yoni-Lingam Worship, 189
yoni mudra, 33, 135, 193, 212, *212*
Yourself Breathing, practice,
    149–50

BOOKS OF RELATED INTEREST

INNER TRADITIONS • BEAR & COMPANY
P.O. Box 388
Rochester, VT 05767
1-800-246-8648
www.InnerTraditions.com

Or contact your local bookseller